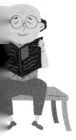
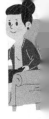

Table

MW01228743

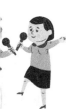

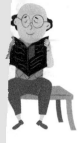
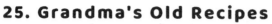

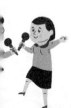
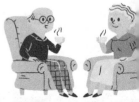

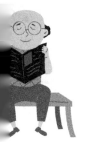
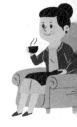

Preface

Dear readers,

We are delighted to welcome you to a special world, a world created for our beloved fellow beings with dementia. This book is not just a collection of stories; it is a lovingly crafted work designed to bring joy, trust, and a sense of connection.

Within this reading book, you will find a series of short stories specifically tailored to the attention span of individuals with dementia. Each story is a little treasure waiting to be discovered and shared. Filled with warmth, humor, and nostalgia, these stories have the power to bring a smile to the faces of your loved ones and fill their hearts with joy.

We firmly believe that stories can play a powerful role in reaching out to those facing the challenges of dementia.

Stories have the gift of touching and moving us; they can make us laugh and remind us that we are part of something greater.

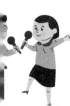

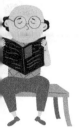
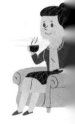

They can evoke memories and create a sense of familiarity and trust, which is crucial for people with dementia.

This book is not just a book, but a journey into the past, a solemn acknowledgment of the present, and a loving embrace of the future. It serves as a reminder that despite the challenges dementia presents, love, joy, and humanity remain possible.

We have crafted this book with the utmost care and dedication, hoping it becomes a source of joy and comfort for you and your loved ones. We trust that these stories will touch the hearts of your dear ones, stimulate their thoughts, and nourish their souls.

With these thoughts, we invite you to join us on this wonderful journey of memory. Let's laugh, cry, remember, and hope together. Let's discover the beauty and power of stories within the pages of this book.

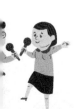
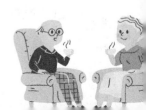

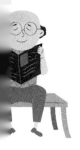
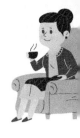

The mysterious diary

It was a sunny afternoon when Emilia found a dusty yet graceful diary in the attic of her old family home. Carefully blowing off the dust from the leather cover, she opened it, and the pages rustled softly under her fingertips. The entries were meticulously written in a fine, yet flowing handwriting that she immediately recognized as her grandmother's. "The mysterious diary of my grandmother," she thought with a smile, sitting down on an old suitcase to read.

The first entry dated back to the summer of 1948. Emilia could almost smell the scent of freshly cut hay and hear the sound of children splashing in the nearby lake as she read her grandmother's vivid descriptions. She read about village festivals where everyone came in their best clothes and danced late into the night. She read about the excitement when the first car arrived in the village and the astonished wonder of the villagers.

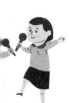
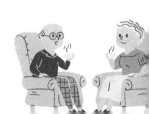

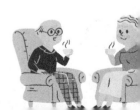

She also read about the simple joys of everyday life: freshly baked bread, Sunday strolls, and the sound of rain on the roof window.

Emilia delved deeper into the stories, experiencing the past through her grandmother's eyes. She read about her grandmother's first love, a young man named Jakob, who enchanted her grandmother with his charm and warm demeanor. She read how they watched the sunset together from the old mill, holding hands and making plans for the future.

She read about the deep sadness when Oliver went to the city to find work and the loving letters they exchanged. She read about the joy of reunion when Oliver returned after years and proposed to her grandmother. She read about the simple but joyful wedding they celebrated in the village, and how the entire village came together in dance and joy. Emilia felt the love that her grandparents had shared, and the warmth of that love filled her heart.

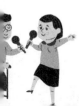

She read about the challenges and joys of building a life together and the birth of her mother. She read about the happy and difficult times her grandparents had gone through together, always with love and respect for each other.

As Emilia closed the diary, she felt closer to her grandmother and her story than ever before. She no longer saw her grandmother just as the dear old lady she had always known but also as the young girl full of dreams and hopes, the strong and loving woman who had led a fulfilling and rich life.

The mysterious diary was a window into the past for Emilia, a way to share the joys, dreams, and hopes of her grandmother. It was a gift of memory that Emilia cherished with a smile on her face and love in her heart. She decided to share her grandmother's stories with her family to keep the memories alive and pass on the love that her grandmother had recorded in her diary. Because, as Emilia realized, memories are the most precious legacy we have.

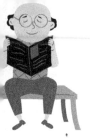
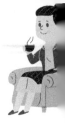

The Search for Clues

Once upon a time, there was a man named Ethan who lived in a small, cozy town at the foot of a green mountain. The town was filled with charming half-timbered houses with beautifully painted shutters, and Ethan knew every corner of it because he had grown up there.

One day, while Ethan was cleaning his attic, he came across an old, dusty wooden box. He wiped off the dust and carefully opened the box. It was full of old family photos, letters, and various trinkets from times gone by.

As he sifted through the box, he found an old map that was partially hidden under a stack of old letters. The map showed his hometown and the surrounding areas, but what caught Ethan's attention was a series of crosses scattered across the map. He recalled that his grandfather had told him stories of lost treasures when he was a little boy. Could it be that the crosses on the map marked these treasures?

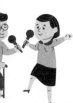
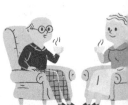

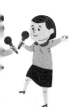
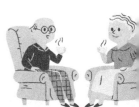

With a smile on his face, Ethan set out to find these supposed treasures. He followed the crosses on the map, leading him to different places in the town, places he hadn't visited since his childhood.

The first cross on the map led him to the old playground where he and his friends had spent countless hours as children. Here, he found a small, rusty toy train that he had lost as a child. As he held the train in his hand, he reminisced about the carefree days when they rode the tracks with their trains and imagined themselves as famous train conductors.

The next cross on the map led Ethan to the lake where he had often gone fishing with his father. Under a rock, he found an old pocket knife that his father had given him. He remembered the warm summer days when they sat by the lake together, casting their fishing lines into the water, and talking about everything and nothing.

Ethan continued to follow the crosses on the map, discovering more and more lost objects from his past.

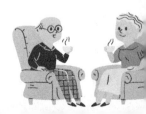

Each find sparked a flood of memories and emotions that made Ethan happy and gave him a sense of satisfaction.

At the end of the day, Ethan returned home with arms full of lost treasures and a heart full of precious memories. He realized that the true treasure hunt was not in the search for material things but in the rediscovery of forgotten moments and feelings that these things awakened in him.

Ethan went to sleep and dreamed of the beautiful memories he had regained that day. And so ended a day full of discoveries and memories, a day that made Ethan happy and showed him how rich his life truly was.

The search for traces was more than just a quest for lost items. It was a journey into the past, a rediscovery of the joy and happiness hidden in memories. And that is the true treasure hunt that each of us carries within.

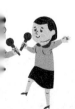

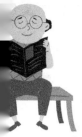
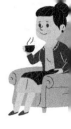

The Magical Music Evening

It was a mild summer evening in the small town by the lake. The sun had just set, and the stars began to twinkle in the sky. A small stage was set up in the town square, and the residents of the town gathered to experience a special evening – the magical music night that took place every year.

Mr. Smith, a friendly older gentleman with silver-gray hair and warm brown eyes, was particularly excited. He had never missed the magical music night. The music always stirred memories of happy times for him and made him feel young and alive.

The first notes of a familiar melody echoed, and Mr. Smith closed his eyes for a moment. It was the song "Black eyes" that he had always loved. The gentle sounds of the violin and the rhythmic clatter of the drums immersed him in thoughts. He recalled a dance evening many years ago when he had danced to this song with his beloved wife, Maria. She had looked so beautiful in her red dress and with her radiant smile.

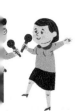
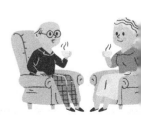

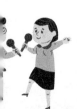
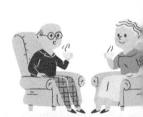

Another song played, "Above the clouds" by Reinhard Mey, and Mr. Smith felt a wave of nostalgia wash over him. He remembered how, as a young man, he had dreamed of becoming a pilot and soaring above the clouds. Although that dream had never come true, he still felt drawn to the freedom and adventure promised by this song.

As the orchestra began to play "Thoughts are free," Mr. Smith couldn't help but quietly hum along. He had often sung this song to his children when they couldn't sleep. It reminded him of the many nights spent comforting his children and telling them stories.

Between the songs, he listened to the stories told by the host – stories about the songs and the artists who had written them. Each story was a small piece of history that made the music even more meaningful.

As the evening came to an end and the last song, a soothing one called "Goodnight, Friends", was played, Mr. Smith felt fulfilled and happy.

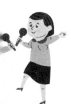

The music had not only provided him with an evening of joy and entertainment but also taken him on a journey into the past when he was young, full of dreams and hopes.

He left the marketplace with a smile on his face and a song in his heart, grateful for the magical power of music that could transport him to places and times he loved. He knew he would look forward to the next musical evening, to the new memories he would create, and to reliving the old ones.

And so ends the story of the magical musical evening, a story that reminds us that music is a powerful force that connects us, evokes memories, and brings us happiness.

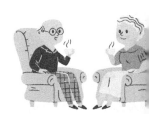

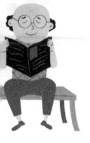
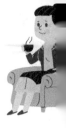

John's Second Chapter

After many fulfilling years as a teacher, John was ready to explore the calmer waters of retirement. He planned to enjoy his golden age with books, gardening, and occasional travels. However, fate had other plans.

John lived in a somewhat run-down neighborhood where many children were disadvantaged due to education budget cuts. He couldn't ignore their misery. He felt that he could still make a contribution, even though he no longer stood in the classroom.

One rainy afternoon, there was a knock on his door. It was little Maria, tears streaming down her cheeks. She couldn't afford tutoring and feared having to repeat the third grade. John's heart broke at the sight of the desperate girl.

An idea began to sprout within him. He could open his home a few evenings a week for free tutoring. He created a flyer and posted it in the local mom-and-pop store. The message spread like wildfire, and soon families from the entire neighborhood came seeking help.

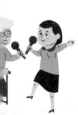
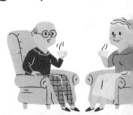

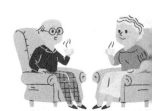

John was deeply moved each time he witnessed the perseverance of his young students who, despite all the challenges, didn't give up. Maria flourished under his encouragement and passed her exams with flying colors.

The word spread, and soon his tables and sofas were filled every evening with eager children. Over the years, John witnessed his students thrive. With each small success, their confidence grew. He couldn't help but beam with pride when Maria became the first in her family to graduate from secondary school. His impromptu school steadily expanded, attracting volunteers who joined the cause.

Although his own children had long since left the nest, John found a new family among the children he taught. Every college acceptance, every wedding, every new job was celebrated —successes achieved through the education he had made possible.

Today, in his eighties, John's small tutoring program has transformed into a well-funded community center. It has positively impacted the lives of hundreds of people.

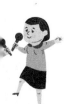

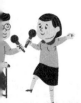

John, still a beloved grandfather figure to all, radiates pride for the doctors, teachers, and business owners who were once his students. John's story is a shining example of how passion and dedication can ensure that no one is left unsupported and without opportunities. His second half of life may have been even more fulfilling than the first. In fact, retirement was just the beginning of a new, meaningful chapter for John.

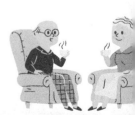

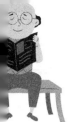
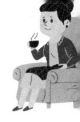

Journey to the Fairyland

Once upon a time, there was a loving person named Hanna who lived in a small, peaceful village. She possessed an extraordinary ability that set her apart from others. Hanna could embark on fantastic journeys within her imagination. One day, she decided to take a trip to a magical fairyland that she hadn't visited since her childhood.

Hanna closed her eyes, and in her imagination, a radiant portal opened. She stepped through and found herself in a fairyland she recognized from her grandmother's stories. The land was as vibrant and lively as she remembered, with shimmering rivers, green meadows, and blooming trees reaching so high they touched the clouds.

Hanna spotted a small, friendly squirrel climbing on a tree trunk. Memories of her childhood days watching squirrels in the park and feeding them nuts flooded back. A smile spread across her face as she recognized this warm moment in her heart.

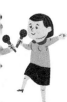
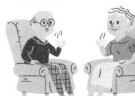

After wandering through the fairyland for a while, she reached a massive castle. She recalled the stories she heard as a child about brave princes and beautiful princesses living in such castles. Hanna entered and was welcomed by a friendly queen who placed a crown on her head. Hanna felt like a true princess, just as she had always imagined as a little girl.

In the castle, Hanna encountered a wise old wizard. The wizard looked at Hanna and recognized her special gift. He showed her how she could fulfill wishes with her magic wand. Hanna remembered how, as a child, she had always dreamed of having magical powers. She wished for everyone in the fairyland to be happy and content. As she waved the wand, a warm, golden light spread across the entire land.

On her journey, Hanna met a friendly dragon. She recalled the heroic stories where brave knights defeated dragons. However, this dragon was not evil; it was friendly and invited Hanna to ride on its back.

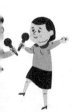

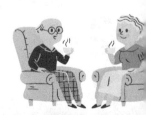

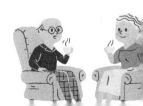

They flew over the fairyland, observing all the beautiful landscapes from above. Hanna felt free and happy, just like when she was a child swinging so high that she felt like she could fly.

Hanna's journey through the fairyland was full of wonderful adventures and beautiful memories. She felt happy and alive, just like in her childhood. When she opened her eyes, she was back in her small village. However, the memories of the fairyland and the joy she had experienced there continued to reside in her heart.

This journey was a reminder of how important it is to keep the child within us alive, to use our imagination, and to appreciate the small joys of life. Because the true fairyland is in our hearts and imagination, waiting to be discovered.

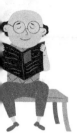
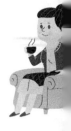

The Pet Adventure

Once upon a time, in a quiet and peaceful small town named Springwood, lived a friendly elderly lady named Mrs. Lewis. Mrs. Lewis had a small, snow-white kitten named Molly. Molly was not just a pet to Mrs. Lewis; she was her best friend and companion.

One morning, as Mrs. Lewis prepared breakfast as usual, she noticed that Molly was missing. She called her name, looked under the bed, behind the curtains, but Molly was nowhere to be found. Mrs. Lewis was concerned and decided to embark on the search for Molly.

She put on her most comfortable shoes, grabbed her walking stick, and set out. The sun was shining brightly, and the sky was covered with fluffy white clouds. She reminisced about the days when she played in the sunshine with her friends as a child. The smile on her face grew with each memory.

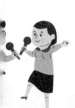
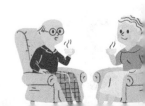

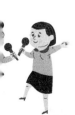

Mrs. Lewis began her search in the park, where she and Molly often took walks. There, she encountered the friendly park caretaker, Mr. Thompson. She recalled the many conversations they had over a cup of tea with Mr. Thompson, who always had the best stories from his youth. Mr. Thompson promised to help in the search and spread the word to others.

The search continued to the bakery, where Mrs. Thompson and Molly often enjoyed the heavenly scent of freshly baked bread. The baker, Mr. Weber, was an old friend. She remembered how she and her late husband used to come to his bakery for Sunday breakfast. Mr. Weber promised to keep an eye on Molly.

Yearningly, she proceeded to the old schoolyard where she used to play with her children. She could feel the laughter and joy in the air, as if time had stood still. She sat on a bench for a while, letting the memories wash over her.

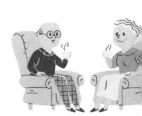

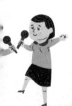
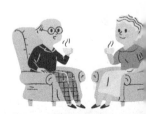

Finally, as the sun began to set, she found Molly in the old barn on the outskirts of town, where she had often played as a child. Molly sat on a hay bale, blinking into the setting sun.

Mrs. Lewis had visited many places and stirred up many memories in her search for Molly. She felt happy and fulfilled. She took Molly into her arms and returned home with a smile on her face. It was an adventure she would never forget.

The story of Mrs. Lewis and Molly shows us that it's not just the destinations that matter but also the journey. Sometimes, unexpected adventures lead us to the most beautiful memories that fill our hearts with joy.

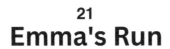

Emma's Run

In the picturesque USA small town of Stonebrook, Emma spent her childhood days. She loved exploring the hidden paths of the nearby forest with her faithful companion, the dog Max. A passionate interest in long-distance running manifested early on, and she dreamt of representing USA at the Olympic Games someday.

However, at the age of 16, Emma began to experience unexplained fatigue. Doctors were puzzled by her mysterious illness. Over time, Emma grew weaker and had to interrupt her high school education. Despite numerous medical examinations, her illness remained inscrutable as Emma's condition fluctuated unpredictably.

During this challenging phase, Emma was supported by her parents and her friend Lucas. With their help, Emma sought to regain her health through rest and gentle walks in the forest. After her recovery, she returned to school and enrolled in the local evening gymnasium, choosing medicine as her focus.

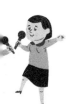

Emma volunteered at a local sports equipment store and learned from experienced coaches. She also joined her school's beginner track and field club. With the support of a coach, Emma kept a training diary and gradually increased her running distance.

When she transitioned to university to study sports science and sports medicine, Emma hoped that her newly acquired knowledge would benefit her recovery. She befriended her university team's running mates, Hanna and Samuel, who imparted valuable insights into nutrition, strength training, and injury prevention.

Qualifying for her first 10k run filled Emma with great joy. Her research focused on chronic fatigue, and she conducted interviews with other patients. She graduated with honors and subsequently worked as a physiotherapy assistant while applying for advanced degree programs.

Emma received acceptance into a prestigious sports medicine program and secured sponsorship from a local sports equipment manufacturer.

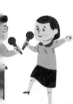

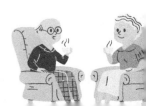

Through intensive training with Hanna and Samuel, who were by then elite marathon runners, she was able to elevate her performance level. Emma qualified for her first Dallas Marathon and received sports drinks specially tailored to her needs.

Emma's master's thesis analyzed blood markers in patients after physical exertion. After graduating as one of the top students in her class, she took a position at an Olympic training center. Her responsibilities included treating elite athletes, monitoring performance data, and creating individual training plans.

Today, Emma participates in marathons purely for pleasure, while managing her own successful physiotherapy practice. Her story exemplifies the power of perseverance, support from others, and holistic approaches to overcoming challenges. She serves as a shining example that one can achieve their dreams despite setbacks and adversities, as long as they have the courage to keep going.

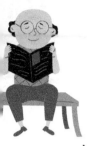
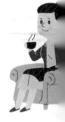

The Imaginary Time Travel

It was a rainy afternoon when Natalie sat on her favorite armchair, gazing out of the window. The drops tapping against the window reminded her of the melody of a long-forgotten childhood memory. She closed her eyes and let the gentle melody carry her to another time.

Suddenly, she found herself on the town square of her hometown, just as she remembered it from her childhood. She could hear the laughter of the market vendors, smell the fragrance of fresh flowers and baked bread. She saw herself as a little girl, joyfully running between the stalls, admiring the vibrant colors and the variety of treats.

Natalie continued to wander through the streets of her past and stood in front of the old school building where she had spent many years. She saw her old classmates with whom she had played and laughed. She saw herself as a teenager, full of dreams and hopes for the future.

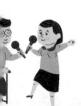
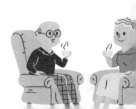

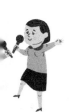
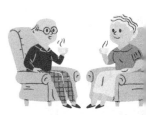

On her journey through time, Natalie also encountered people who had deeply touched her. She saw her first love, a boy with radiant blue eyes and a shy smile. She saw them strolling hand in hand through the park, exchanging their first awkward kisses. She felt the butterflies in her stomach, the excitement she had felt back then.

Natalie continued her journey and encountered her grandmother, a strong and lovable woman who had always supported her. They found themselves in the kitchen, baking cakes together and exchanging stories. Natalie's grandmother hadn't been with her for a long time, but in that moment, she could feel her warm embrace and hear her loving voice.

Eventually, Natalie found herself in the house where she had raised her own children. She saw her kids playing and laughing, and she witnessed herself as a young mother, loving and caring for her children. She felt the deep love and happiness she had experienced in those moments.

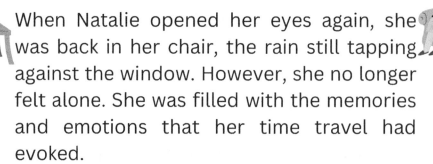

When Natalie opened her eyes again, she was back in her chair, the rain still tapping against the window. However, she no longer felt alone. She was filled with the memories and emotions that her time travel had evoked.

This imaginary journey through time was more than just a trip to the past. It was a reminder of the people and places that had shaped Natalie's life. It was a reminder that, even though life can be challenging at times, it is also full of wonderful moments and beloved people. It was a reminder that, no matter how much time passes, the memories of the people we love and the moments that brought us happiness always stay with us.

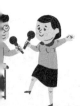

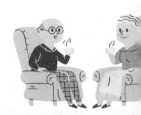

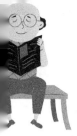
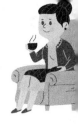

The Lost Wallet

It was one of those magnificent autumn days, where the sky shimmers deep blue, and the foliage glows in the most vibrant colors. Daniel, a spry retiree with a heart for life's small moments, took his daily morning stroll through the park.

While appreciating the beauty of autumn, his gaze fell upon something unusual: an old leather wallet, hidden under a pile of fallen leaves. With curiosity and a hint of excitement, Daniel picked up the wallet and carefully brushed off the leaves.

Inside, he discovered a faded ID card bearing the name Joseph Brown, along with some old business cards and receipts. However, the contact information provided was either illegible or outdated.

Determined to find the rightful owner, Daniel made it his mission to track down Joseph.

He inquired at surrounding shops and cafes, but no one recognized the name or could provide any assistance.

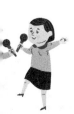
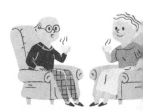

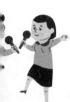

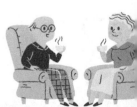

The search seemed fruitless, and Daniel felt discouraged. But he didn't give up. One day, almost having lost all hope, he turned to the local city library. The elderly librarian, who had been living in the town for decades, immediately recognized the name. 'Mr. Brown, isn't it? He lives quite nearby, on Maple Street,' he said, guiding Daniel to Joseph's house.

With renewed hope in his heart, Daniel made his way and knocked on the door of a modest but cozy house. An older man opened the door and looked at him in surprise. When Daniel showed him the wallet and told his story, Joseph couldn't hide his joy. It turned out that this wallet was full of memories - memories of his deceased wife and their shared adventures.

Joseph then invited Daniel inside and offered to share a cup of hot coffee together. They spoke about their lives, their dreams, and the small joys of everyday life. Joseph talked about his love for classical music, history, and travels he had undertaken with his wife. Daniel found a kindred spirit and a friend in Joseph.

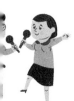

From that day on, no walk of Daniel was complete without a detour to Joseph's, for a cup of coffee and some stories from the past. They discovered common interests and started attending local concerts and exhibitions together. Daniel witnessed how Joseph, who had lived a long time in loneliness and seclusion, blossomed and found joy in life once again.

What started as a simple search for the owner of a lost wallet turned into a deep friendship and an enrichment of both men's lives. Daniel realized that he had not only given Joseph a gift but had also received an unexpected gift himself: a new friendship that enriched his life in ways he never expected.

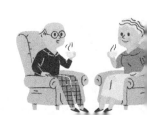

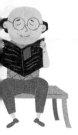
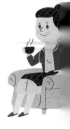

The Living Play

It was a rainy afternoon in November when George entered the old theater in his town. He had come to see a special play performed by his friends and neighbors. George had always been a big fan of theatrical performances, and he was looking forward to an afternoon filled with stories, emotions, and magic.

The play they were performing this time was called "The Magical Play," known for its spectacular costumes, captivating music, and imaginative scenes. It was a tale of adventure, love, courage, and hope, promising to take the audience on an unforgettable journey.

As the lights in the theater dimmed and the curtains opened, George felt his heart beating faster with excitement. The stage was bathed in warm, golden light, and the actors, in their magnificent costumes, looked like characters from another world. The music began to play, and the story began to unfold.

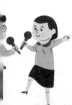

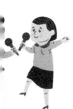

George was immediately drawn into the plot, following the adventures of the heroes, cheering and empathizing with them, laughing and crying along. The performers were so talented and passionate that everything they did felt absolutely vivid and real. It was as if the boundary between the stage and reality had blurred.

Then something incredible happened. Right in the middle of the performance, the stage began to transform. The sets and props came to life, characters stepped out of the stage frame, and moved throughout the entire theater space. It was as if the play itself had become magical.

George couldn't believe his eyes. He saw the heroes and heroines of the play beside him, heard their voices, felt their emotions. He was no longer just a spectator but a part of the story. He experienced the adventures, joys, and challenges of the characters.

This experience meant more to George than just a play.

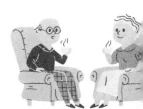

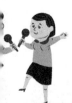
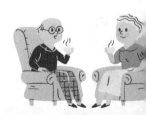

It was a journey into his own past, a recollection of the stories and dreams of his childhood. It was a reminder of the magic of theater, the power of imagination, the joy of sharing and experiencing.

As the play concluded and applause echoed through the theater, George felt fulfilled and happy. He had not only witnessed a wonderful performance but also awakened precious memories and created new ones. He rediscovered the magic of theater and felt the joy of life.

Leaving the theater with a smile on his face and a song in his heart, George knew he would always cherish this day and looked forward to many more magical plays in the future.

The Unexpected Lucky Day

It was a gray and rainy Tuesday morning. Mrs. Jackson, an elderly lady, sat alone at home, staring out the window and feeling somewhat sad. She missed the company, the activities, and the laughter that once filled her house.

Just as she was beginning to lose herself in her sadness, the phone suddenly rang. It was her old friend Hilde, whom she hadn't seen since school days. They chatted for hours about old times, laughed about shared memories, and shared news. The phone call with Hilde brought a smile to Mrs. Jackson's face and brightened her day a bit.

Hardly had she hung up when the doorbell rang. Surprised, Mrs. Jackson opened the door and found a magnificent bouquet of flowers on the doorstep. It was a gift from her granddaughter Lisa, who was studying in another city. The sight of the colorful flowers and the thought of her dear granddaughter brought tears to Mrs. Jackson's eyes.

But the day was not over yet. In the afternoon, a package arrived for Mrs. Jackson. It was a beautifully decorated box, and inside, she found old black and white photos from her wedding.

She hadn't seen these photos for decades and had completely forgotten about them. The pictures brought back beautiful memories of her deceased husband and the wonderful day of their wedding.

In the late afternoon, another surprise awaited her. Mrs. Jackson's son John, who worked abroad, unexpectedly came for a visit. She could hardly believe it when she saw him at the door. They embraced tightly and spent the evening together, talking, laughing, and enjoying their time together.

This day, which had started so sadly, had transformed into one of the most beautiful days in Mrs. Jackson's life. Each surprise had brightened her mood and dispelled her loneliness. She felt loved and appreciated, and she was grateful for the wonderful surprises the day had brought.

The story of Mrs. Jackson reminds us that even in the saddest moments, joy and happiness can be just a moment away. It teaches us that love and affection can come in many forms and that the memories of happy times can help us endure difficult times. It's a story that brings hope and joy.

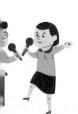
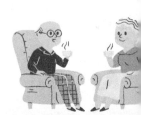

The Birthday Celebration

Once lived a friendly old man named Albert in a small, cozy town. He was known for his radiant smile and kind demeanor. Albert had a special person in his life - his granddaughter Lucy. Lucy was a lively young woman with a heart full of love for her beloved grandfather.

One day, Albert's 80th birthday approached. Lucy wanted to make this special day a memorable experience for her grandfather. She began planning a birthday surprise that would surely bring a smile to his face.

Lucy knew that Albert was a big fan of jazz music. In his youth, he had often danced in jazz clubs and had even toured with a famous jazz band. So, Lucy decided to invite a jazz band to play at Albert's birthday party. She knew that the music would bring him joy and evoke many happy memories. She also started reaching out to old friends and acquaintances of Albert.

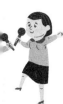

She invited them all to join the celebration and share their beautiful memories of Albert. Lucy wanted Albert to feel how much he was loved and how many people he had touched throughout his life. On the day of the party, Albert beamed with excitement. He didn't know what Lucy had planned, but he was ready to spend the day with his beloved granddaughter. When the music started playing, and Albert heard the familiar jazz melodies, his eyes lit up. He couldn't believe that his beloved music was being played live in his living room!

As one by one, old friends walked through the door, Albert was overwhelmed with joy. He listened to their stories, laughed at old jokes, and even danced to some of his favorite jazz tunes. It was an evening full of laughter, love, and happy memories.

The birthday party was a complete success. Albert couldn't stop smiling about the surprise Lucy had planned for him.

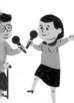

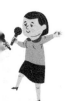

He felt loved and honored, grateful for the beautiful memories he could share with so many people.

Lucy saw her grandfather happy and fulfilled and knew she had done the right thing. She not only provided him with an unforgettable birthday surprise but also gave him the opportunity to celebrate his past and collect even more happy memories.

This story is a reminder that it's the simple things in life—love, friendship, music, and shared memories—that truly make us happy.

It's a reminder of how important it is to honor and appreciate the people in our lives and to celebrate the beautiful moments we've shared with them.

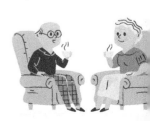

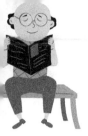
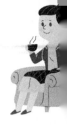

Journey Through the Seasons

Once lived a man named Mr. Brown in a quiet town called Aspen Heights. One day, he decided to embark on an imaginary journey—a journey through the seasons to relive the most beautiful moments from each season of his past.

The journey began with spring. Mr. Brown found himself in a blooming garden. He could smell the aroma of freshly baked bread from his mother's kitchen, as he recalled the bright color palette of flowers in full bloom. He saw himself as a little boy playing with his dog and jumping in puddles left by the spring rain. The joy and laughter from those times filled his heart with happiness and warmth.

As spring transitioned into summer, Mr. Brown found himself on a sandy beach. He could hear the sound of the ocean waves and feel the warm sunlight on his skin.

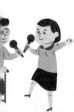

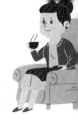

He saw himself as a teenager, swimming with friends and building sandcastles. He remembered the long summer days when they laughed and told stories late into the night. These memories brought a broad smile to his face. Summer gave way to autumn, and Mr. Brown found himself in a forest adorned with colorful leaves. He could smell the scent of damp foliage and freshly baked pumpkin pie. He saw himself as a young man, flying kites with his children and leaping through piles of leaves.

The beauty of autumn and the joy he shared with his children filled his heart with love and gratitude.

Eventually, winter arrived, and Mr. Brown found himself on a snow-covered hill. He could hear the crunch of snow beneath his feet and feel the cold winter air on his face.

He envisioned himself as an older man, sledding and building snowmen with his grandchildren.

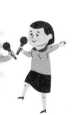

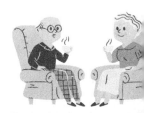

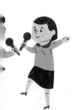
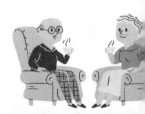

He remembered the delight in their eyes and the laughter that filled the cold winter air. These memories brought tears of joy to his eyes.

At the end of his journey, Mr. Brown felt fulfilled and grateful. He had embarked on a journey through the seasons and through his life. He had experienced the most beautiful moments from each season and every stage of life. He had laughed, cried, and loved. He had awakened memories that filled his heart with happiness and love.

The story of Mr. Brown reminds us that life is a journey through the seasons, full of beautiful moments and precious memories. It shows us that the past is a treasure we carry in our hearts, bringing us joy and happiness. It encourages us to cherish every moment and recognize the beauty of each season and age.

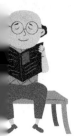
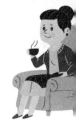

The Mysterious Treasure Map

Once lived in a small village a curious and adventurous boy named Emilio. Emilio loved exploring the forests and fields surrounding his village. One day, during one of his excursions, he stumbled upon an old, weathered treasure map.

The map was covered with mysterious symbols and signs leading to a hidden treasure. Filled with excitement, Emilio showed the map to his best friends, Elena and Max. They were immediately thrilled and decided to embark on a quest to find the treasure.

Their journey took them through dense forests, over high mountains, and through deep valleys. They encountered many challenges and difficulties, but they did not get discouraged. They helped each other, solved puzzles, and stuck together no matter what happened. One day, after many weeks of traveling and searching, they finally arrived at the location marked on the map. It was an old, abandoned cave at the foot of a giant mountain. With pounding hearts and burning anticipation, they entered.

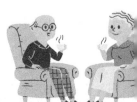

After a while, they finally discovered a large, old chest. They opened it expectantly, but instead of the anticipated gold and jewels, they found something entirely different. Inside the box were old letters, photos, and mementos.

At first, they were disappointed. However, as they began to read the letters and look at the photos, they realized that they had found a completely different treasure. These were memories and stories of people who had lived long ago. They read about love and friendship, adventures and dreams, hopes and fears.

They spent many hours in the cave, reading the letters, examining the photos, and sharing the stories with each other. They laughed, cried, and marveled at the beauty and depth of the human experience.

At the end of the day, they left the cave with hands full of old letters and photos, hearts full of new insights and experiences. They hadn't found a material treasure, but they had found something much more valuable—the memories and stories of people who had lived before them. On the way back to their village, they laughed and shared the stories they had discovered.

They realized that the true adventure was not in the search for treasure but in the memories and stories they had uncovered on their journey. This adventure had bonded them closer together and imparted the valuable lesson that true treasures in life are often not material but reside in the stories and memories we collect and share throughout our lives.

After a while, they finally discovered a large, old chest. They opened it expectantly, but instead of the anticipated gold and jewels, they found something entirely different. Inside the box were old letters, photos, and mementos.

At first, they were disappointed. However, as they began to read the letters and look at the photos, they realized that they had found a completely different treasure. These were memories and stories of people who had lived long ago. They read about love and friendship, adventures and dreams, hopes and fears.

They spent many hours in the cave, reading the letters, examining the photos, and sharing the stories with each other. They laughed, cried, and marveled at the beauty and depth of the human experience.

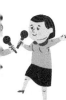
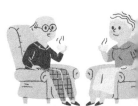

At the end of the day, they left the cave with hands full of old letters and photos, hearts full of new insights and experiences. They hadn't found a material treasure, but they had found something much more valuable—the memories and stories of people who had lived before them.

On the way back to their village, they laughed and shared the stories they had discovered. They realized that the true adventure was not in the search for treasure but in the memories and stories they had uncovered on their journey.

This adventure had bonded them closer together and imparted the valuable lesson that true treasures in life are often not material but reside in the stories and memories we collect and share throughout our lives.

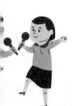

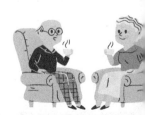

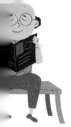
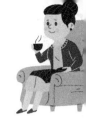

Visit to the Hometown Church

The warm summer sun shone brightly in the sky as Grace strolled through the familiar streets of her childhood town. So many years had passed since her last visit, yet the gentle melody of the past lured her back to these familiar surroundings.

With every step she took on the familiar cobblestone pavement, buried memories came alive again. The scent of freshly baked bread wafting from her mother's kitchen... the click of marbles on the sidewalk as she played a game with her friends... her father's hearty laughter on long summer evenings. A soft smile played on Grace's lips as these memories filled her.

Soon, the old venerable stone church emerged, a testament to time and history. She opened the creaking doors and breathed in the peaceful silence that pervaded the sacred space. The golden sunlight danced through the brightly painted stained glass windows, telling biblical stories and casting a rainbow of colors onto the old wooden benches.

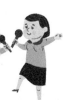
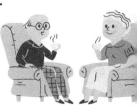

Grace walked along the familiar aisle and took a seat near the front. With closed eyes, she could hear the echoes of past Sunday services and special celebrations. The faces of old friends and beloved ones no longer present illuminated behind her closed lids. A sense of peace and contentment flowed through her.

In this familiar environment, Grace felt the urge to honor her memories. She lit a candle, uttered a quiet prayer, and reflected on the people who had shaped her life. The flickering light and the warmth of the candle created an atmosphere of tranquility and solace.

She sat in silence for a while, getting lost in thoughts and allowing her memories to flow freely. The church had always been a place of community, where people came together to share their faith and hopes. Grace reminisced about joyous weddings, loving baptisms, and dignified funerals that had taken place here. She recalled the comforting words of the pastor, speaking with a gentle voice about love, forgiveness, and hope.

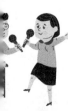

As she rose and continued through the church, Grace discovered that the church held more treasures from her past. She admired the intricate paintings and statues adorning the walls. She marveled at the fine details of the altar and the majestic painting of the crucifixion of Christ. In each detail, she found a connection to her past, to the stories and teachings instilled in her as a child.

Grace sat down once again, letting her gaze wander across the church. The silence of the church enveloped her like a warm blanket, providing her a place of peace and contemplation.

She could feel the presence of all the people who had visited this place before her, who had spoken prayers, sung songs, and lived their own stories here.

After a while, Grace left the church, but she knew it would always hold a special place in her heart. The church was not just a stone building but a symbol of her past, her family, and the community that had once surrounded her.

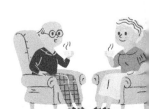

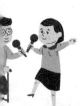
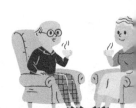

A short walk led her to the town cemetery, surrounded by tall oaks and adorned with colorful flowers. Here, too, she found peace and solace. With a gentle smile, she wandered among the tombstones, pausing here and there to read the name of an old friend or relative.

The tranquility of the cemetery gave Grace a chance to remember the people who had shaped her childhood and youth. She gently ran her fingers over the cool marble slabs, read the engraved words, and reminisced about shared moments. She laid down flowers, lit candles, and whispered quiet prayers.

In the shade of an old oak tree, she sat for a while, gazing at the tombstones, letting herself be embraced by a bit of sadness. It was a sweet-bitter sadness, mixed with gratitude and love for the people who were a part of her life.

After a long, quiet moment, Grace stood up and left the cemetery. She felt calm and fulfilled; a deep connection to her past had accompanied her throughout the day.

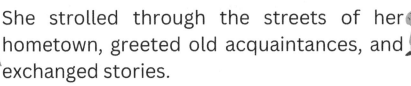

She strolled through the streets of her hometown, greeted old acquaintances, and exchanged stories.

With every step she took through the town, Grace felt more and more at home. She had left the city to lead her own life, but she had also always left a part of herself here. The streets, the buildings, the church, and the cemetery – they all were part of her history, her identity.

As the sun set on the horizon, Grace stood on the hill where she had played as a child, looking at her hometown. The golden rays of the setting sun bathed the city in a soft, warm light.

With a feeling of peace and contentment in her heart, Grace returned to her current home, enriched by the memories and experiences of her visit. She knew that she could always return to her hometown to find solace, peace, and a connection to her past. Her hometown was a part of her, and she was a part of her hometown. It was a connection that would endure beyond time and space.

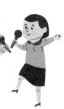
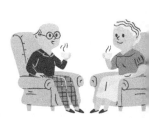

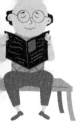
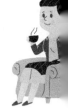

The Wondrous Workshop

In a small, cozy town lived a grandfather named Robinson with his grandson Paul. Robinson was a former craftsman, and Paul, though only ten years old, had a fascination for building and inventing. Their favorite pastime was tinkering and building together in the old garage they had transformed into a workshop.

The garage was filled with a variety of tools, from hammers and saws to screwdrivers and pliers, and each had its own story. Robinson had used these tools for decades and could tell Paul exactly when and how he had built or purchased each one.

Their first joint creation was a simple spinning top. They spent an entire afternoon shaping the wood, sanding it, and polishing it. When they were done, they let the top dance on the garage floor. They laughed and cheered as the top spun faster and faster, celebrating their success with warm cocoa and cookies.

After the spinning top, many more projects followed.

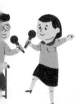
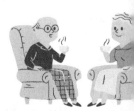

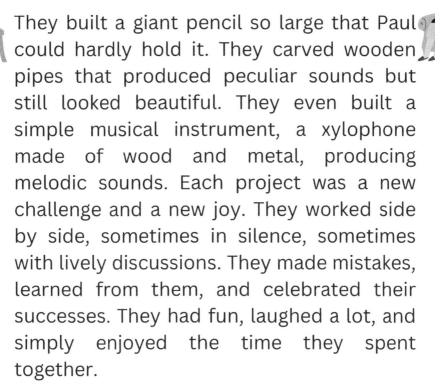

They built a giant pencil so large that Paul could hardly hold it. They carved wooden pipes that produced peculiar sounds but still looked beautiful. They even built a simple musical instrument, a xylophone made of wood and metal, producing melodic sounds. Each project was a new challenge and a new joy. They worked side by side, sometimes in silence, sometimes with lively discussions. They made mistakes, learned from them, and celebrated their successes. They had fun, laughed a lot, and simply enjoyed the time they spent together.

It wasn't just the objects they created that made this time so special. It was the process of creating, the feeling of success, and above all, the sense of community. It was the joy of creating something together and the memories they built in the process.

The garage became a place of creativity and laughter, a place where grandpa and grandson forgot about time and were simply happy. It became a place filled with wonderful objects and even more wonderful memories.

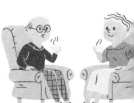

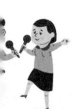

This story is a reminder of the joy and happiness that collaborative creation can bring. It's a reminder that the most important thing in life is often not what we do but who we do it with. It's a reminder that the most beautiful moments are often the simplest - a laughing child, a proud grandfather, a garage full of wondrous objects, and precious memories.

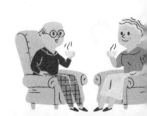

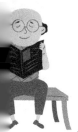
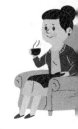

The Apple Harvest

In a small town, surrounded by gentle hills and lush meadows, lived the Jones family. Every year, when autumn arrived and the leaves changed their colors, it was time for the apple harvest in the family's own orchards.

One day, the grandparents, parents, and children all set out together to the apple trees. They carried baskets and ladders, and the anticipation of the harvest made their hearts beat faster.

When they reached the orchard, they were amazed by the variety of apples hanging from the trees. There were green, red, yellow, and even some with a hint of blue. They all hung luxuriously from the branches, waiting to be picked.

As they picked the apples, they discovered a variety they had never seen before. The apples were smaller and had a dark red color. Curious, they tried one and were delighted by its sweet and juicy taste. They decided to collect these apples separately to later make juice from them.

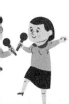
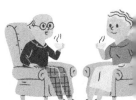

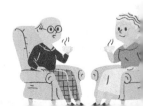

During the harvest, several acquaintances passed by. They were warmly invited to join the harvest and taste the apples.

The children played and laughed while the adults worked and chatted. It was a cheerful and sociable atmosphere. After a few hours, they had gathered enough apples. They loaded their baskets onto an old cart and headed home. Upon arrival, they began preparing apple juice. They used an old but still functional juice press that the grandfather had built many years ago.

While the younger family members pressed the juice, Grandma set out to bake an apple pie. She mixed flour, sugar, eggs, and butter, added the freshly picked apples, and let the cake bake in the oven. The scent of the cake filled the entire house, making everyone hungry.

Finally, the cake was ready, and the freshly pressed apple juice was ready to drink. They all sat together at the table, enjoyed the juice and cake, laughed, and told stories. It was a wonderful day, filled with work, fun, community, and delicious food.

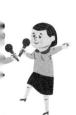

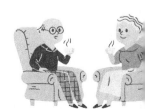

The story of the apple harvest reminds us of the joy that simple activities and coming together with others can bring. It shows us how the discovery of new things and the sharing of experiences can enrich our lives. It is a story that brings joy and warmth, reminding us of the beauty of nature and the joy of community.

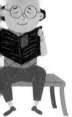

The Own Café

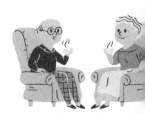

Once upon a time, there was a little girl named Paula who, as if drawn by magic, always ended up in her grandmother's sunlit kitchen. A sweet fragrance lingered in the air, causing her heart to race. Her grandmother, a kind woman with soft wrinkles around her eyes and the warmest smile, was a gifted baker. Every time she dipped her hands into the dough and immersed herself in her magical baking world, Paula played at her feet, observing with wide, amazed eyes.

These moments of childhood left a lasting impression on Paula, igniting a deep passion for baking within her. She dreamed of one day opening her own little café, a place where people could come together over a warm coffee and freshly baked treats.

As Paula grew up, her dream remained alive. After years of learning in various renowned restaurants and refining her baking skills, the day came when she felt ready to pursue her dream. She began searching the picturesque streets of her hometown for the perfect location for her café.

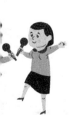

For months, she searched for a suitable place, but every space had its hurdles. However, one day, when she had almost lost hope, she stumbled upon a small, charming building with large windows that, despite its rundown condition, exuded irresistible charm. She felt it in her heart - this was the place she had been looking for.

Paula threw herself into the renovation of this hidden treasure with all her energy. She painted the walls in warm colors, brought in cozy furniture, and adorned the space with loving details. And, of course, there was a large, open kitchen where she could showcase her baking skills.

But the journey was not always easy. Unforeseen repairs got in the way and cost more than her tight budget allowed. In those moments, she thought of her grandmother, of her patience and love for baking. She drew strength from these memories and worked tirelessly.

Finally, the big day arrived. Paula opened the doors of her café, and the scent of freshly baked croissants, crispy scones, and heavenly chocolate cookies filled the air.

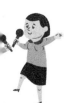
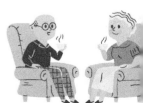

She waited with bated breath for the first guests, but the day passed slowly, and no one entered. But as the sun set and Paula nearly lost hope, the door opened, and an older man walked in. Drawn by the scent of baking, his eyes lit up with joy as he took the first bite of a warm, buttery croissant. He promised to come back and tell others about this hidden gem.

In the weeks that followed, word spread about Paula's café. More and more people streamed in to gather, laugh, and savor the sweet delights. Paula saw her café become a community hub, a place where old friendships were revived, and new ones formed.

Today, Paula's Café is a beloved institution in the town. Everyone who walks in is welcomed by the sweet aroma and the warm atmosphere, just as Paula experienced it as a little girl in her grandmother's kitchen. Despite the difficulties and challenges, Paula has realized her dream and kept the memories of the happy times in her grandmother's kitchen alive.

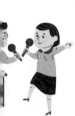
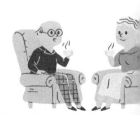

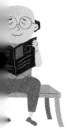
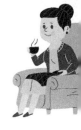

Visit to the Birthplace

In a quiet corner of the world, an old man named Johann lived. One day, he decided to visit his birthplace, a small village he hadn't seen in many years. With a suitcase full of memories and a mix of excitement and nostalgia, he set out on his journey.

As he entered the village, he immediately recognized the old stone bridge under which he used to play as a child. It was still as sturdy and inviting as in his memories. He could still recall throwing stones into the stream beneath the bridge and hearing the splashing they caused. It was as if time had stood still.

He strolled through the narrow streets of the village and rediscovered his old home. It was a bit weathered now, but still as charming as in his youth. He could hear the echo of his mother calling him for dinner and the laughter of his siblings playing in the garden.

On his way, Johann encountered many old acquaintances and friends. He met Mr. Davis, the old baker, who still baked the best bread in the village. He met Mrs. Harris, his first teacher, who had always encouraged him to learn and be curious.

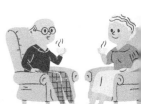

He also met some of his old playmates who were now grandparents themselves. One of the most surprising discoveries Johann made was in the old village school. In a corner of the classroom, he found his old school photo. It was dusty and slightly faded, but he could clearly recognize himself and his classmates. It was a piece of his past he had forgotten, and it brought a broad smile to his face.

The journey was a rollercoaster of emotions for Johann. There were times of joy, times of nostalgia, and times of surprise. But the most overwhelming feeling was that of happiness. He was happy to revisit his birthplace, meet old friends, and rediscover lost memories.

This story is a reminder of the joy and happiness a journey into the past can bring. It is a reminder that the places that shaped us and the people we loved are always a part of us. It is a reminder that finding lost things often means rediscovering lost memories. And above all, it is a reminder that, no matter how much time passes, the joy and happiness we found in the past always live within us.

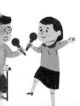
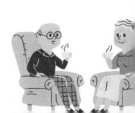

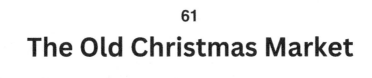

The Old Christmas Market

It was a chilly December evening when Hans, wrapped in a warm coat, crossed the snow-covered streets of his charming hometown. Since the death of his beloved wife Elise, he had avoided the annual Christmas market, a place that was once filled with joyful memories and lovely traditions. The holidays had lost their sparkle, and it was easier for him to stay in the quietude of his home, enveloped in old memories.

However, this evening felt different. An inexplicable force drew him out into the cold, and as he walked, he noticed familiar smells and sounds that stirred a whirlwind of emotions within him. The scent of fresh pine branches and roasted chestnuts permeated the crisp winter air, blending with the distant sounds of laughter and Christmas carols. Memories of happier times, when he and Elise strolled through the market, sampled treats from each stall, and exchanged loving glances, overwhelmed him.

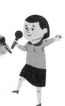
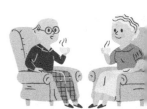

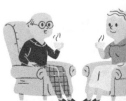

A smile, hidden for years, appeared on his face. As he turned the corner, a shimmering scene unfolded before him, resembling a living painting.

The Christmas market was immersed in a sea of sparkling lights, children played joyfully in the snow, and families browsed the stalls in search of the perfect gift.

It felt so familiar yet so distant.

He strolled from booth to booth, each holding a special place in his heart. Here, he had bought Elise her first gift, a delicate lace handkerchief. And over there, under the densely leafed mistletoe, they had shared their first kiss.

Hans was drawn to his favorite stall by the enticing scents, operated by the always-smiling baker, Mr. Young. His mouth watered as he saw the familiar, warm gingerbread. "A package, please," he said with a voice filled with nostalgia. The baker smiled broadly, remembering Hans and Elise as young lovers who had enjoyed their time together at the stall.

Hans sat on a bench, overlooking the entire market.

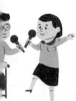

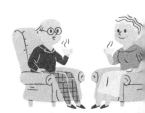

As he bit into a gingerbread, his gaze fell upon a little girl with rosy cheeks building a snowman. She reminded him so much of his daughter when she was little. A wave of warmth flowed through him, and his heart felt lighter. He knew that despite Elise's absence, the holidays had come alive again. Their love and the spirit of Christmas would continue to live on in his heart, in the memories they had created together, and in the new memories he would still create.

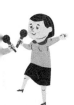

The Circus Visit

Felix sighed contentedly as the rusty old station wagon came to a stop in front of the impressive circus tents. Decades had passed since his last visit as a young boy. As he stepped out of the car, the sights and sounds transported him back to a happier time.

Walking through the entrance, a wave of nostalgia overwhelmed Felix. The scent of popcorn and cotton candy wafted through the air. Colorful banners fluttered above them, accompanied by carousel music. His grandchildren squealed with joy, pulling at his hands.

The circus director welcomed them with a dramatic gesture. "Welcome to a magical night under the big circus tent!" As the crowd cheered, Felix felt like a wonderstruck child once again.

The acrobats were the first to perform, catapulting themselves through the air as if weightless. Felix recalled a similar performance from his youth, warming his heart.

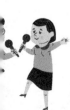
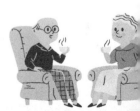

Then came the clowns, with their slapstick antics that brought laughter to both young and old alike. Just like in the past, their pie-throwing and stumbling lifted his spirits. The animal performances followed - lions and tigers leaped through rings of fire, elephants balanced on colorful balls. Felix watched captivated, reminiscing about bringing his own children here. Trapeze artists soared high above, defying gravity with daring tricks.

During the intermission, the crowd mingled at games of chance. Felix spotted an old friend from school days running a throwing booth. After a playful reunion celebration, he threw a ball, dunking the man in water amid laughter.

As the second half commenced, motorcycle stunt riders raced inside the ring, narrowly avoiding each other by a hair's breadth. Then came the riders, performing a beautiful equestrian display to music. However, the grand finale truly took Felix's breath away. A parade of all the acts circled the ring together, earning applause and cheers.

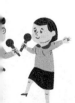
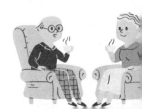

Confetti rained down, and balloons soared into the sky, bringing smiles to both young and old alike.

As they stepped out into the night, Felix turned to his family with a grateful smile. "Thank you for this journey into my memories. I haven't felt this happy in years." The magic of the circus had lifted his soul and reminded him of brighter days.

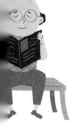
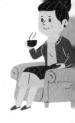

Gabriel's Memory Journey

Gabriel stepped slowly onto the paved path to the train station, lost in thought. He had seventy-five eventful years behind him – years mostly filled with happiness and contentment in his humble farmhouse, alongside his beloved wife Elise. However, since her death, the days had become quieter and lonelier.

As he reached the station, a steam train was pulling in. The familiar sight and the hiss of steam reminded him of times gone by. A smile crossed his face as he boarded the train and took a seat by the window.

With the rhythmic clatter of the train, his mind began to wander into the past. He recalled their first meeting at a dance in the village community hall. Elise had enchanted him with her radiant smile and sparkling eyes. They were shy but determined to get to know each other. The furtive glances, the awkward smiles, and the first tentative conversations – all of it laid the foundation for their lifelong love.

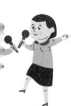
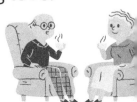

Gabriel didn't realize when he slipped into a light sleep. When he opened his eyes, the landscape had changed. The snow-covered fields had given way to a dense forest. A movement in the corner of his eye caught his attention. Two deer were gracefully moving through the trees.

This tender sight brought memories of Elise to life, who was equally gentle and loving. He closed his eyes and delved deeper into his memories. The images of their wedding day came to mind—a radiant day, Elise in her simple yet beautiful dress. The deep love in their gazes as they said "I do" before the altar. The subsequent years on the farm, the shared work in the fields, the cozy evenings by the fireplace. The birth of their sons, the joy and pride he felt seeing Elise with the children.

A jolt brought Gabriel back from his memories. The train had arrived. He disembarked hesitantly and glanced at the platform. His heart skipped a beat. There stood Elise, radiant and young as on the first day.

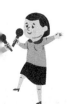

Gabriel was confused and stammered, "But how...?" Elise just smiled and lovingly stroked his cheek. "Come, my love. Our anniversary celebration awaits us."

Before he could grasp it, he found himself in their cozy farmhouse, surrounded by their sons and grandchildren who laughed and shared stories. His heart swelled with joy. At the head of the table sat Elise, her loving smile brightening the room. In that moment, Gabriel realized that this was not a dream. It was a gift, a memory showing him that Elise would always be with him, in his heart and in the stories and memories they had written together. Their love would always remain alive, in him and in their family.

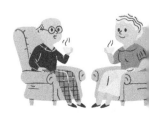

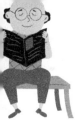
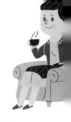

A Cozy TV Evening

It was a cold winter evening in the small town where Grandma Emma and Grandpa Karl lived. Their children and grandchildren had decided to prepare a special surprise for them. They planned a TV night where they would all watch their favorite shows from the past together.

The family arrived early in the evening, bringing popcorn, chocolate, and other treats. Grandma Emma and Grandpa Karl were overjoyed to have all their loved ones around them. They had no idea what the evening had in store for them.

After dinner, everyone gathered in the living room. The television was turned on, and the first show began - it was "Dalli Dalli," one of the most popular game shows of the 70s and 80s. Grandma Emma and Grandpa Karl were surprised and delighted. They reminisced about the many evenings they had watched the show together. They laughed at the old jokes and played along with the quiz game. It was a true delight to remember those beautiful times.

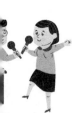
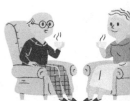

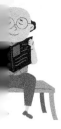

The next show was "The big prize," another popular quiz show. Grandpa Karl shared stories of how he always tried to answer the questions before the contestants did.

They all played along and enjoyed the excitement and fun of the game. Then came 'The Dream Ship,' one of Grandma Emma's favorite series. She recalled the exotic locations and romantic stories. She told her grandchildren about the different countries and cultures she had discovered through the series.

Finally, the evening ended with a special surprise - an episode of 'Little House on the Prairie,' a series the whole family loved. They watched the episode, laughed, and cried together. They exchanged memories of the characters and stories they had cherished so much.

It was a beautiful evening filled with laughter, joy, and memories. Grandma Emma and Grandpa Karl were overjoyed. They had enjoyed their favorite shows, traveled back in time, and spent precious time with their family.

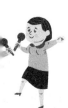

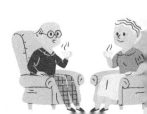

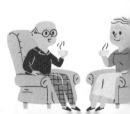

This TV evening was more than just a simple night in front of the television. It was a journey into the past, a shared experience that brought them all closer together. It was an evening that showed them that the most beautiful moments in life are often the simplest - to laugh, remember, and love together.

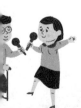

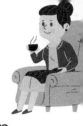

Grandma's Old Recipes

It was a sunny Saturday morning when Grandma Sophia revealed the secret of her old, traditional recipes to her granddaughter Lisa for the first time. Lisa, a passionate young chef, had been eagerly waiting to learn more about the dishes she had loved since her childhood. Grandma Sophia opened her old, worn-out cookbook and showed Lisa the first recipe: 'Grandmother's Potato Soup.' She explained that the recipe came from her own grandmother and included special ingredients that are hardly known today, such as parsnips and lovage. While they gathered the ingredients, Grandma Sophia shared stories from her childhood, when she helped her mother in the kitchen and learned the recipe for the first time.

They laughed a lot as they peeled and chopped the potatoes and vegetables. Lisa loved hearing her grandma's stories and learning the old cooking techniques.

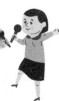

Both of them were happy and enjoyed the time together in the kitchen. As the soup finally simmered on the stove, Grandma Sophia showed Lisa another old recipe: 'Mom's Apple pie.

She explained that the dough had to be rolled very thin and that the most important thing was the filling - apples, raisins, cinnamon, and sugar. As they prepared the dough and sliced the apples, Grandma Sophia told Lisa stories of the many Sundays when she enjoyed this delicious Apple pie with her family.

Suddenly, the kitchen door opened, and Grandpa Benjamin walked in. He smiled as he saw Grandma Sophia and Lisa in the kitchen and asked if he could show them his favorite dish. It was an old recipe he had learned from his grandfather: "Grandpa's sour ribs." He explained that the secret of the recipe lay in the marinade - vinegar, mustard, onions, and spices.

As they prepared the ribs, Grandpa Benjamin told Lisa stories of the many evenings he spent in the kitchen with his grandfather cooking this dish.

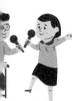
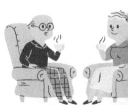

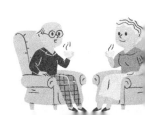

The kitchen was filled with laughter, stories, and the delicious scent of Grandma's potato soup, Mom's apple strudel, and Grandpa's sour ribs. Grandma Sophia, Lisa, and Grandpa Benjamin enjoyed their time together in the kitchen, the memories they shared, and the joy of cooking old, traditional recipes. They looked forward to tasting the dishes and discovering more recipes and stories from the past.

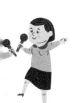

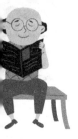
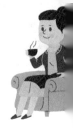

The Power of Laughter

It was an ordinary morning when Alfred, a friendly older gentleman, made an extraordinary discovery. Alfred was known for his sense of humor and infectious laughter, but on this day, he was about to uncover an even deeper truth about the healing power of laughter.

Alfred's adventure began at his favorite café. While enjoying his morning coffee, he witnessed a group of children attempting to rescue a cat from a tree. The children were making the wildest and funniest movements to reach the cat, and Alfred couldn't help but laugh. It was a hearty, joyful laughter that warmed his heart and swept away all worries.

Next, Alfred went to the market. There, he observed a vendor struggling to catch his unruly chickens. The chickens fluttered in all directions, and the vendor stumbled and comically tripped over his own feet.

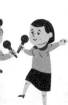
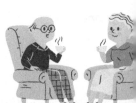

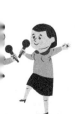
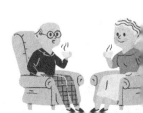

Once again, Alfred burst into laughter, and this time, other market-goers joined in. It was a wonderful feeling to share the joy and laughter with others.

Later in the day, Alfred encountered his old friend George. George was known for his amusing stories and jokes, and on that day, he had some particularly good ones in store.

They laughed so hard that tears filled their eyes, and they could barely catch their breath. It was a laughter that emanated from deep within and filled every cell in their bodies with joy. By the end of the day, Alfred felt more alive and happier than ever before.

He had experienced the healing power of laughter and the joy and happiness it could bring into his life.

He had learned that laughter is not just a reaction to something funny but also a way to celebrate life and recognize the beauty and humor in everyday situations.

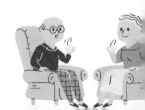

From that day forward, Alfred made a commitment to laugh every day and share the joy of laughter with others. He realized that laughter is a language everyone understands, a medicine everyone needs, and a gift that everyone can share.

As a result, Alfred was not only loved for his laughter but also for his wisdom and kindness. He brought joy and light into the lives of those around him and became a shining example of the magic and healing power of laughter.

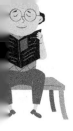
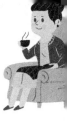

The Book of Magical Pictures

Once upon a time, there was a friendly elderly gentleman named Jakob, who lived in a cozy house on the outskirts of a tranquil village. One day, while cleaning his attic, he came across an old, dusty suitcase. Curious, he opened the suitcase and found an old picture book inside, which he hadn't seen since his childhood. The book was filled with colorful illustrations and wonderful stories that reminded him of long-forgotten times.

Oliver settled into his favorite chair, opened the book, and let his eyes glide over the first pages. The images leaped out of the book and seemed to move before his eyes. Suddenly, he felt drawn into the stories, as if he were a part of them himself. The first story was about a brave knight on a mission to rescue a princess from the clutches of an evil sorcerer. Oliver could recall how, as a little boy, he had loved such adventure stories.

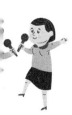
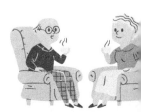

He could almost feel the wind in his hair as he imagined the knight riding through the landscape on his horse. A smile spread across his face as he revived these memories. The next story told of a beautiful mermaid living in a sparkling ocean.

Jacob remembered how fascinated he was as a child by the stories of the sea and its creatures. He could smell the salt in the air and feel the waves on his skin as he immersed himself in the tale. Another chapter depicted life in a bustling medieval market. Jacob recalled the joy he felt as a young man trading in local markets. He could almost hear and smell the bustling activity, people's laughter, and the scent of fresh bread and spices. The last chapter portrayed a peaceful scene in a forest, filled with animals living together in harmony. Jacob reminisced about his youth, taking long walks in the woods and savoring the chirping of birds and rustling of leaves. He could feel the cool forest air and the tranquility of the woods as he looked at the images.

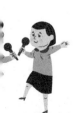
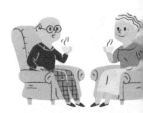

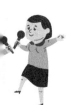

Jacob's journey through the picture book was like a trip through his own past. Each story stirred precious memories and emotions within him. As he closed the book, he felt a deep sense of satisfaction and joy. The book had given him the opportunity to dive once again into the wonderful stories and experiences of his past. This story illustrates that the past never truly disappears; it lives on in our memories and in the stories we tell. The magical picture book was a valuable gift for Jacob, helping him relive his memories and awaken joy in his heart.

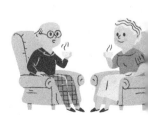

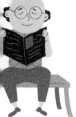

A Visit to the Flea Market

Once there lived a friendly gentleman named Emilio in a quiet, small village. Emilio was known for his love of flea markets, and it was one of his favorite pastimes to wander through the stalls in search of hidden treasures. One sunny Sunday morning, Emilio set off for the old flea market on the edge of the village. He was looking forward to the day and was eager to see what treasures he would discover. He arrived at the flea market and was immediately greeted by the familiar mixture of sounds and smells - the soft murmur of voices, the clinking of dishes, and the sweet aroma of fried sausages and fresh coffee. Emilio began his tour of the flea market, strolling from stall to stall. At one of the stalls, he discovered an old chessboard. As he picked it up, he was immediately reminded of the countless hours he had spent playing chess with his grandfather as a child.

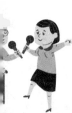

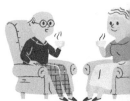

He could still vividly remember his grandfather teaching him the moves and strategies. With a happy smile, Emilio bought the chessboard. Emilio continued on to another stall, where he stumbled upon an old crate of vinyl records. As he sifted through the collection, he came across a record from his favorite band from his youth. He remembered the concerts he had attended and the feeling of freedom and rebellion that the music had stirred within him. Emilio felt filled with warmth and nostalgia as he purchased the record.

Eventually, Emilio reached a stall with a collection of old books. One particular book caught his attention - an old fairy tale book that looked just like the one his mother used to read to him as a child. As he opened the book, he could smell the familiar scent of old paper and ink, and suddenly he was once again a little boy, captivated by his mother's stories. With a feeling of gratitude, Emilio bought the book.

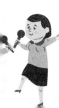

As Emilio left the flea market, he was filled with joy and gratitude. Each of the items he had purchased had stirred up memories and emotions within him that he had long forgotten. He understood that the true treasures at a flea market are not the items themselves, but the memories and stories they evoke within us.

Emilio returned home and carefully placed his new treasures around his house, where they would remind him of the beautiful memories they had stirred within him. Each visit to the old flea market was a journey into the past for Emilio, an opportunity to rediscover the joy and happiness hidden within his memories. And that was the true value of the treasures he had found at the flea market.

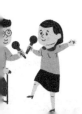
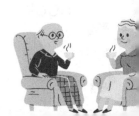

The Old Beech Tree

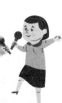

It was a cool autumn day in the small village of Maplewood. John sighed as he placed another log on the dwindling woodpile. Winter was approaching, and he didn't know how he would keep his family warm without more firewood. They led a simple life, unfamiliar with wealth, but they always had enough love and unity.

As he picked up another branch, he noticed movement. An old tractor had driven down the narrow dirt road and now stopped in front of their property. A weather-beaten man stepped out and nodded to John. "Good day. My name is Owen. I heard you could use some assistance."

John hesitated, his pride making it difficult for him to accept help. But the cold reality was that they did indeed need help. He reached out his work-worn hand. "Thank you. I'm John. John remembered his own climbing adventures in the branches of these beech trees as a boy. "Look, Papa!" Elena called out as a flock of sparrows swooped down to feast on the beech nuts.

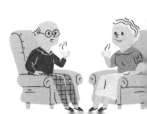

Elena and Anna laughed cheerfully as they watched the squirrels frolicking among the leaves. John smiled as he saw their carefree joy.

Soon, the woodpile was tall and complete again. But Owen hadn't done enough yet. "I'll bring you a hot stew tonight. No one should go hungry in winter." John wanted to protest but stopped himself - the man's generosity was a gift he should gratefully accept.

As the evening fell and the sky painted itself in warm hues, Owen returned with a lavish meal. His stew simmered in an old enamel pot. Fresh farmer's bread and crisp apples filled a basket. But best of all was the surprise Owen had brought - a bag of sugar cubes to sweeten the hot cocoa.

The girls' eyes sparkled as they stirred the sweet addition into their warm cocoa. Owen told stories that fascinated them all, of adventures in distant lands and magical beings that appeared at twilight.

John contributed his own stories, and soon they all laughed until their bellies ached with joy.

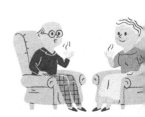

As the flames danced, John saw faces from the past around the fire - his mother singing old folk songs, his grandfather carving wooden toys. Love, friendship, and community seemed never to truly fade when kept in the heart. Weeks passed, and Owen became a permanent part of the family's life. He helped with repairs, brought meals, and shared his wisdom and stories. On Christmas Eve, as the snow gently fell, they gathered around their candlelit Christmas tree. There were no material gifts, but their hearts were full of gratitude and joy. They had learned that life's true gifts are not material but are found in the precious moments of friendship and love. So they warmed themselves with the joy and the community that would carry them through all the seasons to come.

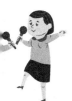

Gabriel's Travel Companion

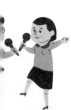

It was a rather cool autumn day when Gabriel boarded the train with a deep sigh. He prepared for a long journey, his only companions being his solitary thoughts and the view of the passing landscape through the train window.

The trees, dressed in their colorful autumn attire, seemed to gaze at him sadly as the train slowly departed the station.

Several stations later, as the train stopped and passengers boarded and disembarked, Gabriel noticed a small dog hesitantly entering the carriage. Its fur was matted, and it looked thin and frightened. Gabriel, who in his younger years always had a soft spot for strays, immediately felt pity for the little creature.

"Come here, little one," he called gently, patting the spot beside him. The small dog approached cautiously, almost as if expecting a blow.

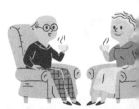

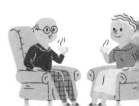

Gabriel reached out his hand, allowing the dog to sniff his scent. Slowly, the dog's tail began to wag.

Gabriel pulled out the sandwich he had packed for the journey and tore off a small piece for the dog. Its eyes lit up with joy and gratitude.

While the dog enjoyed nibbling on his bread, Gabriel stroked his ears and felt less alone for the first time in a long while.

"What shall we call you, hmm?" he asked the dog, smiling. The little dog licked Gabriel's hand as if to give his approval.

In the hours that followed, Gabriel began to tell the little dog stories from his life. Stories from his childhood on the farm, his time as a baker, and his wonderful life with his beloved wife Elizabeth.

The little dog seemed to hang on his every word, laying his head in Gabriel's lap and sighing contentedly.

As Gabriel spoke, he pulled out the remainder of his sausage bread to share with his new friend.

But to his surprise, he found that the little dog had found a fallen cookie from another passenger under the seat! Gabriel laughed as the little dog proudly placed the cookie in front of him. "You're a clever boy! How about the name 'Jack'?"

That evening, as dusk fell, Gabriel took Jack for a walk along the tracks. Under a sky illuminated by stars, Jack suddenly darted off and returned proudly with a stick twice his size. "Well then, you're my 'Jack Frisbee' from now on!" laughed Gabriel.

When they finally reached their destination, Gabriel felt sad that their journey together was coming to an end. But at home, he had an idea. "Would you like to meet the neighbors, Jack?" he asked the dog. Jack barked happily and wagged his tail. At Gabriel's house, Jack enchanted all the neighbors with his gentle and friendly nature. Perhaps, Gabriel hoped, he had not only found a companion but also a new beginning.

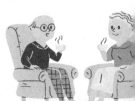

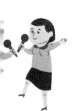

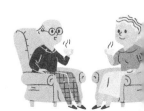

Over time, Gabriel and Jack became inseparable. They took long walks through the fields and forests, now ablaze with the most beautiful autumn colors. Gabriel taught Jack Frisbee many tricks and was rewarded with wet kisses. In the evenings, snuggled up by the crackling fireplace, Gabriel read Jack Frisbee from his old travel books and dreamed of future adventures with his faithful friend.

The Old Letterbox

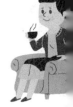

As Gertrudis rummaged through the dusty boxes in her attic, she stumbled upon an old, worn leather suitcase brimming with letters. Her arthritic fingers trembled with excitement as she pulled out the first letter - it was an old letter from her dear mother, whom she hadn't seen in decades.

The elegant, flowing handwriting of her mother transported Gertrudis back to her childhood. She could vividly hear the gentle tone of her mother's voice as if she were standing right beside her. Tears welled up in Gertrudis's eyes, both from sorrow at the loss of her mother and from joy at rediscovering this piece of her history.

Deep within the suitcase, amidst yellowed envelopes, she found letters from old school friends, filled with adventures and mischief, notes passed clandestinely during class, and lovingly written birthday and holiday cards. Reading these words, the faces and voices from Gertrudis's past seemed to come back to life.

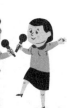
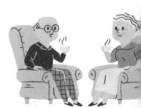

One of the envelopes contained a lovingly written letter addressed to "My dearest Gertrudis" in a bold, distinctive handwriting unfamiliar to Gertrudis. She pulled out a yellowed newspaper clipping announcing the wedding of her aunt Helga, who had passed away before Gertrudis's birth. The letter spoke of hopes and dreams for a happy and prosperous future.

As the darkness of the evening set in, Gertrudis's creaking joints signaled it was time to take a break. But the next morning, refreshed and renewed by a good night's sleep, she resumed her nostalgic journey of discovery.

More letters brought back forgotten memories - of pen pals from the war years, of secret love letters during her courtship with Bernhard, and of lovingly decorated cards celebrating the births of her children.

A letter, addressed in a shaky handwriting, made Gertrudis pause - it was from her old neighbor, Mrs. Weber. At the end of the letter, she found Mrs. Weber's phone number, unchanged after all these years.

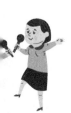
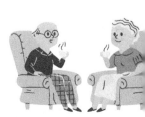

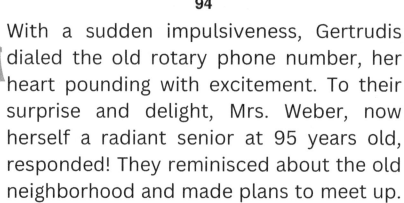

With a sudden impulsiveness, Gertrudis dialed the old rotary phone number, her heart pounding with excitement. To their surprise and delight, Mrs. Weber, now herself a radiant senior at 95 years old, responded! They reminisced about the old neighborhood and made plans to meet up. From there, Gertrudis began reaching out to other individuals whose letters she had rediscovered.

The reunion with old friends injected new vigor and joy into Gertrudis's days. They shared memories, laughed over old photos, and savored a cup of hot tea while rekindling their once-lost connections. Despite the changing world around them, their friendships remained steadfast and unbreakable.

These lost letters served as a bridge that reconnected Gertrudis with people, places, and moments she thought were lost forever. In rediscovering her history, she found joy, connection, and a renewed sense of belonging.

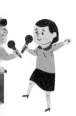

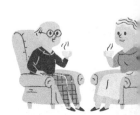

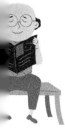

A Past Love Story

It was a dreamy afternoon in the small town of Fernwood. The sun gently shone through the windows of Mrs. Carter's house, a kindly elderly lady. She sat in her favorite armchair, surrounded by photos of her loved ones, and gazed at a special picture lying on the table beside her. It was an old black and white photo of a young man with sparkling eyes and an infectious smile. This picture sparked a flood of memories in Mrs. Carter; it was the image of her late husband, Mr. Carter. The two had met many years ago in a dance class. Mrs. Carter still remembered vividly the first dance they had shared. It was a slow waltz, and they had fit together like magic. Every movement, every step was in perfect harmony, and she felt like she was on cloud nine. She recalled looking into his eyes and knowing that she had found the man with whom she wanted to spend the rest of her life.

Their days together were filled with laughter, love, and adventure. She remembered their walks in the park, their picnics by the river, and their travels together.

Each moment was like a precious treasure in her memory. She remembered their wedding, a simple yet beautiful occasion, surrounded by family and friends. And she remembered the vow they had made to each other: "For better or for worse, until death do us part."

But it wasn't just the big events she remembered. It was also the little things that filled her heart with joy. Like Mr. Carter making her coffee every morning, how he brushed the hair from her face when they talked, or how he always called her 'my darling.' Over the years, they had faced many challenges together and had grown stronger and closer. Even though Mr. Carter was no longer with her, she could still feel his presence in every room of her house, in every song she heard, and in every old photo she looked at.

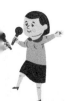
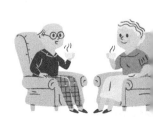

Mrs. Carter let her eyes wander over the photo and smiled. The memory of their love story, of the happy times and the lifelong bond they shared with Mr. Carter, was like a warm blanket enveloping her. She felt comforted and loved, even when she was alone. She understood that true love never dies; it lives on in our hearts and memories, never truly leaving us alone.

And so she sat there, in her cozy armchair, letting the sweet memories of their forgotten love story come alive again. Every memory, every thought brought a smile to her face and filled her heart with love and warmth. And she knew she would never forget this story because it was a part of her, a part of her life and soul.

Happy Grandpa Johannes

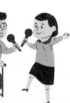

Johannes sighed, his gaze fixed through the window on the misty sky. Life had dealt him a harsh blow; his beloved wife had passed away, and since then, the world seemed less vibrant, the days indistinguishable. Yet one morning, as Johannes stared out the window as usual, the silence was broken by children's laughter and excited voices.

On the neighboring property, belonging to a children's home, he saw children playing joyfully. A thought began to take shape in his mind. At the children's home, Johannes was warmly welcomed by the home director, Mrs. Young. "We can always use helping hands. The children would surely appreciate an extra grandfather," she said with a friendly smile. Johannes' heart raced at the thought.

From that day on, the children's home became his daily destination.

Initially, the new environment felt unfamiliar and he felt unsure, but the bright eyes and infectious laughter of the children quickly dispelled any doubts.

He read to them from old fairy tale books, helped with crafting paper airplanes, and played tag with them in the garden. With every child's laughter, every small hand reaching out to him, long-buried memories resurfaced. Memories of the time when his own children were small and he played with them in the park. Among the children was a small, shy girl named Elena, who formed a special bond with Johannes. Like a delicate flower opening its petals, Elena began to slowly confide in him. When she was teased by the other children because of her stuttering, Johannes found the right words to convey to them the importance of compassion and understanding. Each hug from Elena at the end of the day gave Johannes a sense of belonging and purpose that he had long missed.

On Johannes' birthday, the children surprised him with a lovingly crafted card and a chocolate cake baked by Sra. Young. They sang a serenade for him, and for a moment, Johannes felt young again, surrounded by his growing family of children who loved and cherished him.

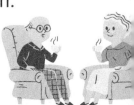

His heart filled with more love than he could have ever imagined. Although the fog of dementia was still present at times, Johannes no longer felt so lost within it. He had found new joy in the laughter of the children, who awakened old memories and enlivened his spirit. In the children's home and in the small hands that eagerly greeted him every morning, he found a reason to enjoy each day anew and to celebrate life.

One day, a new boy arrived at the home, a small, fearful boy named Valentin. Johannes took him under his wing and helped him settle into the children's home.

They spent many hours together, playing chess and reading stories. Valentin reminded Johannes of his own son when he was still young. He felt responsible for the little boy and was determined to help him navigate this new environment.

Over time, Valentin became more confident and began to make friends with the other children. He was no longer the fearful, withdrawn child he once was. Valentin had transformed into a cheerful, lively boy who enjoyed life in the orphanage.

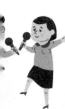

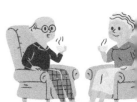

Witnessing this change, Johannes felt a deep sense of fulfillment and joy.

Thus, despite the fog in his mind, Johannes found a new sense of purpose. He discovered that happiness often lies in the simplest things: in a child's laughter, in the joy of winning a game of chess, in the warmth of a hug. And although he knew that the fog of dementia could return one day, he was grateful for these moments of clarity and joy that life in the orphanage provided him. On a beautiful autumn day, when the leaves were glowing in the brightest colors and the scent of roasted chestnuts filled the air, Johannes took the children to the nearby park. They played hide and seek among the trees, collected colorful leaves, and told each other stories.

Johannes felt alive and happy. He saw his own youth reflected in the radiant faces of the children and felt connected to them.

In the evening twilight, as the sky painted itself in the most beautiful colors and the first stars began to twinkle, Johannes sat with the children on a bench and told them about his wife.

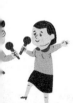

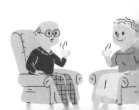

He spoke of their love, their shared adventures, and their family. The children listened intently, empathizing with him. They understood that they too were part of his family, and Johannes felt safe and loved within the community of the orphanage residents.

Over time, Johannes became an integral part of the orphanage. He was no longer just the "extra grandfather"; he was a friend, a confidant, and a teacher. He gave the children love and security, and in return, received joy and hope. He found a new family in the children and a new home in their hearts.

Johannes' story shows that happiness often lies in the simplest things: in a child's laughter, in a walk in the park, in a hug at the end of the day. It demonstrates that it is never too late to find new happiness and that every moment of life is precious. It is a tale of love, friendship, and hope that inspires each of us to embrace life to the fullest and to see each day as a new adventure.

A Stroll Through the Forest

It was a bright, sunny morning as little Jonas and his beloved Grandpa Karl set out into the forest that lay on the edge of their small village. Grandpa Karl, a sturdy elderly gentleman with a warm laugh and eyes sparkling with zest for life, was a great lover of nature. He had often told Jonas about the adventures he had experienced as a young boy in this forest.

As they wandered through the woods, Grandpa Karl showed Jonas the various types of trees and plants. They saw tall firs and gnarled oaks, beneath whose shade moss and ferns spread. They discovered wild raspberries and blackberries, and Grandpa Karl told Jonas how he had collected them as a child and processed them into delicious jams.

Suddenly, they heard rustling in the bushes. They approached cautiously and discovered a small rabbit family playing in the grass. Jonas' eyes lit up with excitement, and Grandpa Karl quietly explained to him the importance of not disturbing the animals in nature.

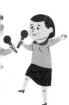
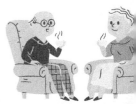

Further into the forest, they came upon a large clearing where deer and stags peacefully grazed. With eyes filled with wonder, Jonas observed the grace and beauty of these animals, while Grandpa Karl told him stories of the many evenings he had spent as a young man watching these majestic creatures in their natural habitat.

As they ventured deeper into the forest, they discovered a mysterious cave. Initially, Jonas was a little fearful, but his curiosity and adventurous spirit prevailed. With Grandpa Karl by his side, they ventured into the darkness. Inside the cave, they found ancient rock drawings telling stories from times past. Grandpa Karl explained to Jonas that these signs could have been left by the region's indigenous inhabitants. It was like an exciting history lesson right in the middle of the forest.

On their way back, they heard the joyful chirping of birds, and Grandpa Karl showed Jonas how to recognize the different bird calls. Jonas was fascinated and promised to bring a notebook next time to write down all the bird calls they had heard.

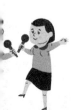
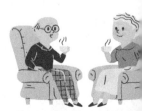

When they finally arrived home, they were tired but happy. This day in the forest had been an unforgettable experience for Jonas, and Grandpa Karl was just as thrilled. They had shared adventures, admired the beauty of nature, and created memories that would last a lifetime.

This story of Grandpa Karl and Jonas' excursion into the forest is a tale of discovery and adventure, reminding us that we are never too old to learn new things and to appreciate the wonders of nature. It's a story that reminds us that the most beautiful memories are often the simplest ones—the time spent with the people we love and the experiences we share with them.

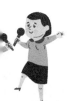

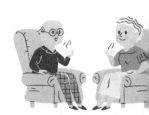

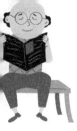
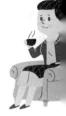

The First Time at Sea

In the small, idyllic town of Pinecrest lived Mr. and Mrs. Young, a lovely elderly couple, in a cozy house on the edge of the forest. Despite their many years, they had never seen the sea. So, they decided to fulfill their dreams and finally take a trip to the seaside.

With packed suitcases and radiant faces, they boarded the train that would take them to the coast. The journey was long, but the anticipation was stronger. They shared stories from their youth and laughed together as they admired the passing landscape.

When they finally reached the sea, they were overwhelmed by the vastness of the ocean and the sound of the waves. They could hardly believe the salty smell in the air and the feeling of the sand under their feet. They walked hand in hand along the beach, enjoying the sight of the sunset.

The next day, they went on a boat trip. They stopped in the middle of the sea, cast their fishing rods, and waited patiently. Mr. Young finally caught a big fish, which made them both laugh. They jumped into the sea and swam together.

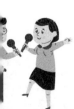
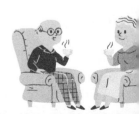

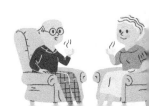

They felt the cool water on their skin and laughed with joy. On the third day, they went on a submarine ride. They were fascinated by the beauty of the ocean, the colorful corals, the shiny fish, and the mysterious sea creatures.

They saw dolphins jumping alongside the submarine, and a turtle swimming leisurely through the water. They were reminded of the many animal books they had read to their children. Every evening, they went to a local restaurant and enjoyed delicious seafood dinners.

They reminisced about the many meals they had cooked together and exchanged stories about their favorite recipes. They savored the local music and even danced to some songs.

They took trips to nearby islands, hiked under palm trees, and collected shells on the beach. They saw birds they had never seen before and admired the beauty of nature.

They recalled the many hikes they had taken in their hometown. At the end of their journey, they felt fulfilled and grateful. They had gathered many new memories and rekindled old ones.

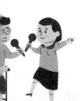

They had seen the sea, swam, fished, and discovered all the wonders of the ocean. They had laughed, danced, and admired the beauty of nature together.

The journey of Mr. and Mrs. Young shows us that it is never too late to pursue our dreams. It reminds us that life is full of surprises and adventures, and that the memories we collect are the most precious treasures we possess.

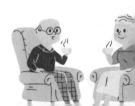

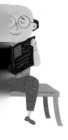
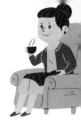

The Melody of Happiness

On a bright and sunny Thursday morning, a bus full of lively schoolchildren, members of the school choir, brought the joy of music to the "Sun yard" senior home. Under the guidance of their musical mentor, Mrs. Smith, the children were filled with anticipation and excited energy to perform their latest songs for the residents.

As they entered the large communal room, they quickly set up their music stands and began to warm up their voices.

The initial notes of the melodies filled the room, rousing the residents from their daydreams. The music created a vibrant atmosphere that brought the seniors to life.

In one corner of the room, Mabel, a former ballerina, began to tap her foot to the rhythm of the music.

She reminisced about the days when she danced to a similar love song from 1944 with her beloved husband. Her eyes lit up, and a faint smile crept onto her face.

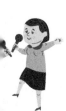
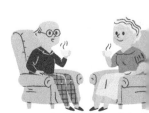

Across from Mabel sat Harold, a former opera singer, who hummed along to the melody in rhythm. He placed his hand on his heart and closed his eyes, completely lost in the music. Mrs. Smith, noticing his obvious delight, signaled to him and encouraged him to contribute his voice. Harold, initially hesitant, eventually let his deep baritone flow into the choir, filling the room with harmony.

When the last piece was played, many residents sang and clapped along, their faces beaming with joy. The choir received standing ovations and enthusiastic calls for an encore. However, since time was short, the children had to promise to return the next week to sing more songs.

And so it became a beloved tradition. Every Thursday, the children brought new songs and melodies to the nursing home. The residents eagerly anticipated these musical visits, which warmed their hearts and stirred up memories.

Over time, deep friendships formed between the residents and the choir members.

Smiles became brighter, conversations livelier, and excitement grew with each visit. One day, even a spontaneous dance party broke out when the choir played a particularly lively big band piece.

The joyful serenades of the choir became a staple of life at the "Sun yard" nursing home. They brought joy and cheer to the hearts of both residents and students alike, demonstrating the wonderful power of music to lift spirits and unite communities. They served as a constant reminder that music, laughter, and community are the best remedies for the soul, regardless of age.

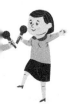

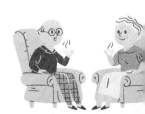

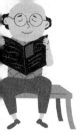
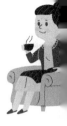

Reunion of an Ancient Love

In a small town once lived Henry and Madison, a couple who were once inseparable. But fate tore them apart, and for several years Henry had been living in isolation in a facility at the other end of the country. Madison remained behind in the house they once called home.

One day, while flipping through old photo albums, Madison came across pictures of her and Henry in their younger years – happy times filled with love and laughter. A feeling of longing took hold of her, and she decided to visit Henry.

After a long journey, Madison finally arrived at the facility where Henry lived. As she entered the room, Henry immediately recognized her. His eyes lit up, and a broad smile spread across his face. They embraced, and in that moment, time seemed to stand still.

They spent the afternoon telling each other stories from their past.

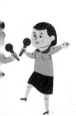
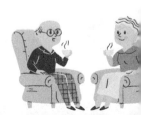

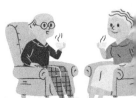

Henry spoke of the years he had spent in isolation, and Madison spoke of her life in the empty house. They reminisced about the happy times they had spent together and the challenges they had overcome. Their stories were filled with love and warmth, and they laughed and cried together.

As the sun went down, Madison made a proposal. She wanted Henry to come back with her to their old home. Henry was surprised but also overjoyed. They decided to spend the rest of their lives together, just like in the old days.

Back in their old house, they began to rebuild their lives. They dusted off old furniture, hung up pictures, and filled the house with love and life. They cooked together, took walks, and enjoyed the simple pleasures of life.

There were also challenges. They had to adapt to new routines and learn to deal with the limitations of old age. But they were happy. They had each other, and that was all that mattered. Their story is proof that love knows no bounds.

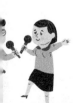
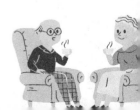

Despite the years and distances that separated them, Henry and Madison found each other again. They remembered the love they had once shared and let it come alive again.

They spent the rest of their days together, telling stories, laughing, and sharing their love. Their story is a reminder that it is never too late to find each other again and that true love always prevails.

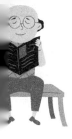
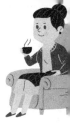

Childhood Feathered Friend

It was a sunny afternoon at the "Rainbow Land" kindergarten in a small village in USA. Little Karl discovered a delicate, brown bird that had hidden itself among the green bushes of the playground. The bird seemed weak, almost fragile, and its tiny eyes looked fearfully at the world around it.

Curiosity overcame Karl's natural shyness. He couldn't just watch the little creature in distress. He decided to help it, and thus began a beautiful friendship.

The next day, Karl packed an extra snack - a few crumbs from his delicious sandwich. With calm and cautious steps, he approached the bird and spoke gently to it, so as not to scare it.

By the end of the week, the little bird had gained enough trust in Karl to eat from his hand. It was a magical moment that filled the little boy's heart with joy. Every morning before class, Karl brought small treats for the bird and softly sang songs while they sat together in the grass.

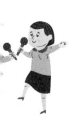
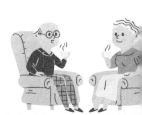

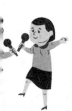
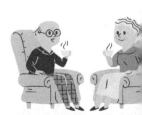

A deep bond of trust formed between the unlikely friends. But one day, Karl noticed the bird trembling and seeming breathless. With careful hands, Karl protected the fragile creature and hurried to Nurse Madison. She was known for her kindness and patience and had often helped the children when they got hurt. Madison carefully examined the bird and thought that rest and good food could help it. Following Madison's instructions, Karl nursed the bird with mealworms and kind words until it regained its strength. The relief Karl felt when the bird was healthy again was indescribable.

As the bird grew stronger again, Karl built it a cozy nest and played gentle imitation games with it. Soon, the bird was singing its beautiful song again, and it was music to Karl's ears. The day the bird could fly again and flew into freedom from Karl's hand was a day of bittersweet joy.

Since then, Karl started coming to the kindergarten earlier every day, bringing snacks for birds and squirrels.

He lovingly cared for injured animals, and his friends saw how important animals were to Karl. They began to share his passion for nature and learned a lot about the animals around them.

Although his feathered friend now lived in freedom, he would forever remain in Karl's heart. Every time Karl saw a brown bird in the sky, he thought of his friend and smiled. He knew that his friend would always have a special place in his life.

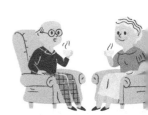

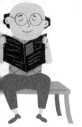
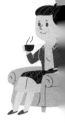

Lost Letters

Jakob sat at the rustic kitchen table with a heavy sigh, sorting through the mounting reminders. The relentless flood of bills - electricity, mortgage, credit cards - seemed never-ending. His job at the local wood factory was on the line due to an impending closure, and the weight of financial hardship bore heavily on his shoulders.

"What are we going to do, Jakob?" Maria asked, a hint of desperation in her voice. Their small farm, which had been in Jakob's family for generations, was at stake. The thought of losing their home was unbearable.

Just as Maria uttered these worried words, there was a knock at the door. It was Anthony Schmitt, the manager of the local bank. "I'm truly sorry, Jakob and Maria. But if you can't pay by the end of the month, I'll have to initiate foreclosure." His words hung heavily in the air as he left the house.

The next few days were bleak and oppressive.

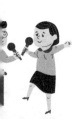
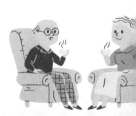

Jakob scoured their finances, searching for solutions, but it seemed futile. Even selling their livestock and equipment wouldn't cover the massive debt. As the end-of-month deadline approached, everything seemed lost.

One evening, while Maria was leafing through an old diary, a small, faded piece of paper fell out. It was a lottery ticket, almost expired, which they had forgotten they had even bought. "Jakob, look at this!" exclaimed Maria, her voice filled with surprise.

Jakob took the lottery ticket and began comparing the numbers with the results of the past weeks out of pure curiosity. His heart raced faster as he realized that the numbers matched. They had won - and it wasn't a small win, but a huge jackpot! In that moment, all their troubles seemed to vanish. The next day, Jakob rushed to the bank with the lottery ticket and triumphantly placed it on Anthony's desk. "Anthony, I think we have a debt to settle!" Anthony's eyes nearly popped out of his head.

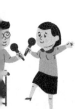
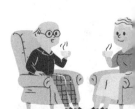

With their newfound wealth, Jakob and Maria first paid off their farm debts and all other obligations. Their relief was immense, but Jakob had an even bigger idea - why not help others who were also in need?

They began supporting their fellow human beings. They donated money to renovate the old community center, bought a new ambulance, and helped families in need.

For the volunteer fire department and even sent anonymous checks to people in financial difficulties. Their generosity knew no bounds and was only surpassed by their humility. The news of their good deeds spread throughout the city. Smiles returned to the faces of people who had experienced so much hardship and difficulty. And for Jakob and Maria, the greatest gift was giving hope to others, just as unexpected happiness had given them a fresh start. In the following weeks, they continued to find forgotten lottery tickets, letters with good news, and other small miracles in their old books and drawers.

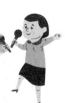
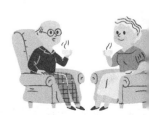

Each time, these discoveries reminded them of how unexpected luck had changed their lives and motivated them to continue doing good. And so ends the story of Jakob and Maria - a tale of the power of hope, the significance of community, and how sometimes the greatest wonders come in the smallest envelopes.

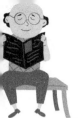
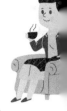

A Day in the City

In a small, peaceful town lived a loving grandmother named Martha. Martha lived alone in a charming old house that she had built with her late husband.

Her only daughter, Anna, lived with her family in a city not far away. One beautiful morning, Anna decided to visit her mother and spend a day with her in town.

Anna picked up Martha, and together they set off for the town. They strolled through the bustling streets, past the colorful shops and the lively marketplace. Anna bought her mother a colorful scarf that matched Martha's bright blue eyes perfectly.

Martha told Anna stories from the past, when she had walked these streets as a young girl. After their stroll through the town, they made their way to the city park.

The park was full of life - children were playing on the playground, couples were strolling hand in hand, and a street musician was playing a cheerful melody on his violin. Martha and Anna sat down on a bench and watched the activity.

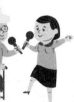
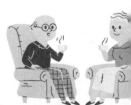

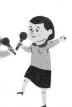

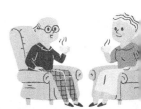

They ate ice cream and laughed at the cheerful ducks swimming in the nearby pond. Suddenly, Martha recognized an old friend whom she hadn't seen in years.

The two ladies warmly greeted each other and exchanged news. It was a joyful reunion that filled Martha with happiness. After visiting the park, Martha and Anna went to a cozy café in the city.

They sat by a window and ordered coffee and cake. As they ate, Martha told Anna about her memories of the café - how she and her husband had spent their first dates here and how they had brought Anna here when she was still a little girl. They talked for hours, exchanging stories and reminiscing about old times.

Anna listened fascinated as Martha recounted her youth, the dances she had attended, the friends she had made, and the adventures she had experienced. As the day came to an end, Martha and Anna drove back home.

They were both happy and fulfilled by the memories and stories they had shared.

For Martha, it was a valuable reminder of old times, and for Anna, it was a precious connection to her mother and her past.

This day in the city was more than just a simple outing. It was a journey into the past, a rediscovery of the joy and happiness hidden in memories. And that's the true beauty of memories - they can connect us, make us happy, and remind us of who we are and where we come from.

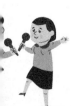

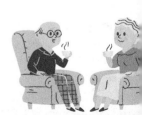

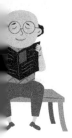
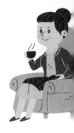

The Museum Visit

In a quiet corner of an art museum sat an older lady named Rosalind on a bench, gazing at a particular painting. It was a large, vibrant artwork painted many years ago by a dear friend. She remembered the first time she saw it, and how it had captivated her with its beauty and energy.

The painting depicted a beautiful summer day in a lush garden. It was filled with lively colors - the rich green of the leaves, the radiant blue of the sky, the lush red of the roses. The colors were so intense that Rosalind could almost smell the scent of the flowers and feel the warmth of the sun on her skin.

The shapes in the painting were equally captivating. There were winding paths that meandered through the garden, and a variety of flowers and trees, each with their own unique shapes. There were also people - children playing, couples strolling, elderly folks sitting on benches, all enjoying the beauty of the day.

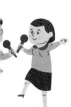
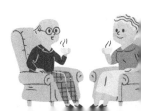

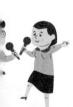
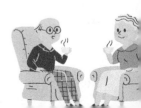

Rosalind let her thoughts and emotions be guided by the colors and shapes of the painting. She remembered the many summer days she had spent in similar gardens. She recalled the joyous laughter of children, the carefree delight of play, the sweet moments of sharing with friends.

She remembered the love she had experienced in her life - the tender love of her parents, the passionate love of her husband, the gentle love of her children. She recalled the challenges and joys of life that had shaped her into the person she was today.

She also remembered her friend, the artist who had created the painting. She remembered his passion for art, his joy in creation, his care for every detail. She remembered the many hours they had spent together, talking about art, life, and love.

Looking at the painting was like a journey into the past for Rosalind. It stirred many memories and emotions in her, allowing her to view her past from a new perspective.

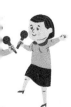

It helped her to recognize the beauty and significance of her life and to appreciate the many people and experiences that had shaped her.

The magical artwork was more than just a painting for Rosalind. It was a mirror of her soul, a window into her past, a source of inspiration and joy. It was a precious treasure that she would always hold in her heart.

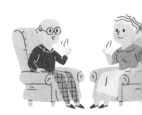

The Promise of the Rainbow

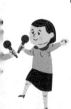
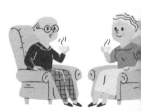

Deep darkness and an relentless storm enveloped the small farmhouse on the edge of the little USA town. The venerable farmer Joseph sat by the window of his parlor, observing the chaotic weather. With every thunderous roar, he flinched, as thunderstorms had always frightened him.

As the storm subsided and the clouds finally parted, Joseph spotted a shimmering arc on the horizon. Sunbeams broke through the clouds, and a colorful rainbow stretched majestically across the sky. It was a sight that took his breath away. As a child, he had often tried to find the end of this fantastic phenomenon.

A memory came to him. His dear mother, who always whispered to him with a loving smile, "Rainbows are a promise, my dear. They mean that the storm is over and better days are coming." Those words had comforted him then and did so again in this moment. With newfound courage, Joseph stood up. He had sat in his house for too long, letting his fears rule over him.

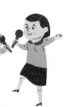

But the rainbow, this messenger of hope, sparked a desire for change within him. He went to the stable and saddled his faithful mare, Lotti. "Let's go, my old girl, for one last adventure," he whispered into her ear. They rode through the vast fields, Joseph following the path of the rainbow. As the vibrant colors finally began to fade, he noticed something glittering in the grass. Upon closer inspection, he discovered a gold nugget embedded in the earth!

With gleaming eyes, Joseph held the gold nugget up to the sun. All his life he had dreamed of finding a treasure, but lacked the courage to seek it. This golden gift, brought by the rainbow, was a sign - his stormy days were over. From now on, he would follow his dreams, no matter what happened. And if dark times were to come, he would only seek the bright promise of hope in the sky.

The news of Joseph's discovery quickly spread throughout the small town. Soon, the residents flocked to his farm, hoping that the rainbow held more gifts in store.

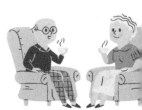

Joseph, once a reclusive man, suddenly found himself amidst a community of friends. They worked together, digging for possible treasures, laughing and singing together. Of all the gold they had hoped for, they found nothing. But the true treasure they discovered was friendship.

In the midst of the cheerful group, Joseph noticed one woman in particular - the charming Emma from the local grocery store. Despite his shyness, he gathered the courage to ask: "Emma, my dear, may I accompany you home after this shared search?" Her radiant smile was answer enough.

Joseph and Emma became inseparable, and soon they were often seen strolling together. In Joseph, courage for another great quest grew once more - he asked Emma if she wanted to be his wife! She said yes, and so the rainbow brought not only gold but also love and a new beginning for Joseph and Emma. And the community learned that true wealth does not lie in gold or material things, but in people and in the love they share with each other.

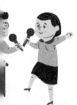
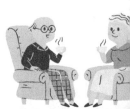

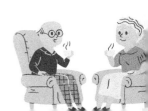

Thus, this story ends with the promise of the rainbow - a promise of hope, love, and community. And the knowledge that after every storm, a rainbow awaits, and with it the chance for a new happiness.

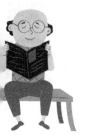
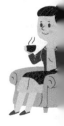

Adventure in the Mountains

Once lived a grandfather named Joseph, who was a passionate mountain hiker and nature lover. One day he decided to take his young grandson Lucas on a hike into the mountains. Lucas, a curious and adventurous boy, was thrilled by the idea.

They packed their backpacks with provisions and set off early in the morning. The first rays of sunlight crept over the mountain peaks as they rode the cable car up the mountain. Lucas's eyes sparkled with excitement as they ascended higher and higher, and the landscape below them grew smaller and smaller.

Upon reaching the top, their hike began. They followed a trail that wound through dense forests and over green meadows. Joseph showed Lucas how to recognize animal tracks and identify the songs of birds. They discovered a beehive in an old tree trunk and watched as the busy bees buzzed back and forth. Joseph was also knowledgeable about herbs.

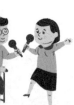
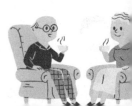

He showed Lucas how to recognize different types and how to gather them for tea. They found thyme, chamomile, mint, and many others. Lucas was fascinated by the diversity and beauty of nature. After a while, they reached a breathtaking mountain lake. The water was so clear that they could see the bottom. They sat by the shore, ate their lunch, and enjoyed the peace and beauty of the place. They even saw a few fish dancing beneath the water's surface. During their hike, they also discovered a variety of flowers. Joseph knew a story about each flower, and Lucas listened eagerly. They saw rare mountain flowers and colorful butterflies fluttering from flower to flower.

As the day drew to a close, they made their way back. They were tired but happy. They had seen and learned so much. The hike was an adventure they would never forget.

Back home, they sat down with a cup of tea made from the collected herbs and shared the stories of the day. They laughed, they shared, and they enjoyed each other's company.

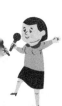
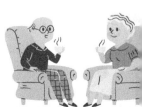

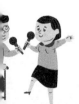

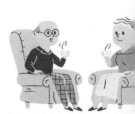

It was a wonderful day, full of discoveries and joy.

This story highlights the beauty of nature and the joy that a shared hike in the mountains can bring. It reminds us of the value of these shared experiences and how much we can learn from nature. It's a story that evokes memories and brings joy.

Rediscovered Father

On a golden autumn day, I drove along the long gravel road that led me to a place I had never seen before. After a long search, I was finally on my way to meet the man I had never met - my biological father. What would he look like? What would he be like? With a deep breath, I stepped out of the car.

Before me stood a stately yet cozy farmhouse. I saw a tall, broad-shouldered man working in the field. His sandy hair was now streaked with gray, but his kind blue eyes were unmistakable. How many times had I gazed at them in the old photos my mother kept? "Dad?" I called out hesitantly.

He looked up, surprised, and dropped his tools. "Paul?" We stared at each other for a moment, taking each other in. Then he approached me and enveloped me in a big, warm hug. "My son, it's so good to see you!" I returned the hug, feeling tears welling up in my eyes.

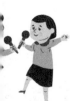

This man, this stranger - he was my father. He led me into the house and called out, "Emily, look who's here!" A sturdy woman with a friendly face emerged, wiping her hands on her apron.

"Oh, is that our Paul?" She hugged me tightly. "I'm so glad you've finally found your way to us, my dear nephew."

Confused, I looked back and forth between my father and Emily. "Emily is my sister," my father explained. "She's your aunt and has always been there for me when I was young and inexperienced."

Emily smiled warmly and squeezed my hand. "We've always loved you and hoped that one day you would find your way to us. You're a part of our family, Paul."

Over a lovingly prepared dinner, my father - Johann, as he wanted to be called - told his side of the story. "I was just a boy when I met your mother. I panicked when she told me she was pregnant. I ran away like a coward." Regret filled his eyes as he spoke.

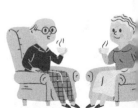

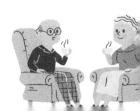

But Emily placed her hand on his. "Now, Johann, there's no point dwelling on the past. What matters is that Paul is here now. We are a family, and we will stick together."

In the following days, Johann showed me around the farm and introduced me to the animals by name.

We worked side by side, repairing fences and making hay bales. Emily was always there to support us and surround us with her loving nature. It felt as though the lost years were being reclaimed. In the evenings, we sat by the fire while Johann told exciting stories from his youth. Emily laughed heartily and occasionally added her own memories. The bond between siblings was obvious, and I felt blessed to be part of this family. As the time to say goodbye approached, Johann's eyes were moist. 'Stay in touch, you hear?' he said with a husky voice. I nodded and hugged him one last time. 'I'm glad we found each other, Dad.

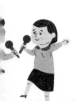

And Aunt Emily, thank you for welcoming me as part of your family.' In that moment, it truly felt that way. A lost father was a found father, and an aunt had found her place in my heart. Our story had just begun, and I knew that from now on, I would be surrounded by a family that loved me unconditionally.

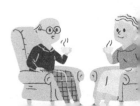

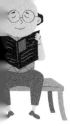
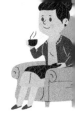

A Night with Grandma and Grandpa

In a small, picturesque town called Brookside lived Grandma and Grandpa Smith, a lovely elderly couple who spent quiet evenings with their beloved grandchildren. Every Friday evening was a special occasion when the whole family gathered to eat, drink, and most importantly, to play board and card games. On this particular Friday evening, one could feel the laughter and excitement in the air. Grandma Smith had prepared her famous recipes: a delicious potato soup for dinner and her special cookies for dessert, served with vanilla wafers. Everyone sat together at the dining table, eating, drinking, and telling stories.

After dinner, it was time for the games. Grandpa Smith brought out the board and card games. There was a variety of games to choose from: Nine Men's Morris, Checkers, "Sorry!", Skat, and Uno. Everyone had their favorite game, and everyone had a chance to win.

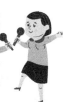
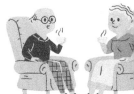

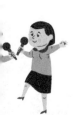

First, they played Nine Men's Morris. Grandpa Smith was an experienced player, but his grandchildren were clever and quick. There were many unexpected twists and funny moments. In the end, the youngest grandchild won, which made everyone laugh.

Afterwards, they played "Scrabble" (really put everyone's language skills to the test.). It was a heated game with many humorous situations. Grandma Smith was thrown out of the game several times, which made everyone laugh. But she didn't give up and eventually won the game.

They also played a round of Chess. Grandpa Smith was the winner, but the grandchildren quickly learned and promised that they would win next time.

To conclude, they played poker. It was an exciting game with many unexpected twists. Everyone had a chance to win, but in the end, it was the eldest granddaughter who emerged victorious.

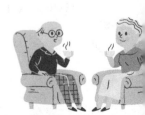

At the end of the evening, everyone went to bed happy and satisfied. They had laughed, eaten, and played. They had created new memories and refreshed old ones. They had spent a wonderful time together and were already looking forward to the next Friday evening.

The story of Grandma and Grandpa Smith reminds us that life's simple pleasures are often the most beautiful. It reminds us that being together with family, laughing, playing, and sharing meals creates valuable memories that last a lifetime. It shows us that happiness is often found in the smallest moments.

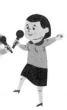

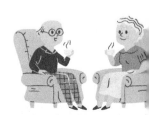

Farm Excursion

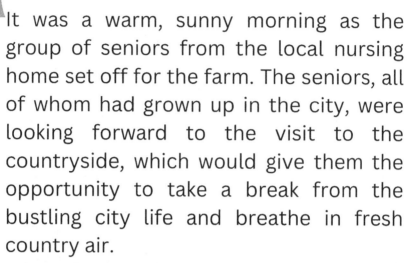

It was a warm, sunny morning as the group of seniors from the local nursing home set off for the farm. The seniors, all of whom had grown up in the city, were looking forward to the visit to the countryside, which would give them the opportunity to take a break from the bustling city life and breathe in fresh country air.

When they arrived at the farm, they were warmly greeted by Farmer Martin and his wife Hanna. They were a friendly couple who had been running the farm for many years and were proud to be able to show the seniors rural life.The day began with a tour of the farm.

They saw cows, pigs, and chickens, and Farmer Martin patiently explained the tasks involved on a farm and how important this work is for the city's supply. The seniors were fascinated by the animals and the workings of the farm, marveling at the contrast to city life.

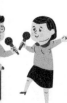
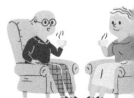

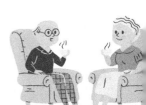

After the tour, each senior was allowed to take on a task. Some fed the animals, while others helped in the vegetable garden. They experienced how much work goes into a farm, while also enjoying the simple pleasure of getting their hands dirty or being close to the animals.

For lunch, Hanna had prepared a festive farmer's meal. There were fresh vegetables from the garden, homemade bread, and a hearty soup. As they ate, the seniors exchanged stories from their childhood, many reminiscing about similar experiences on their grandparents' farms. It was a joyful meal, and the memories and stories filled the space with laughter and warmth.

In the afternoon, they took a walk through the surrounding fields. They watched as the wheat swayed in the wind, as the bees flew from flower to flower, and as the birds circled in the sky. They enjoyed the peace and beauty of nature and felt a deep gratitude for this day.

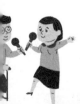

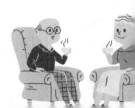

As the day came to an end and they made their way back home, they felt refreshed and fulfilled. They had not only glimpsed into country life but also awakened cherished memories and created new ones. They had laughed, worked, and eaten together. They had experienced the simplicity and richness of rural life and were grateful for it.

The visit to the farm was more than just an outing; it was a journey into the past and a reminder of how important it is to appreciate the simple things in life. It was a reminder that happiness is often found in the simplest moments - in working with your hands, in community with others, and in the beauty of nature.

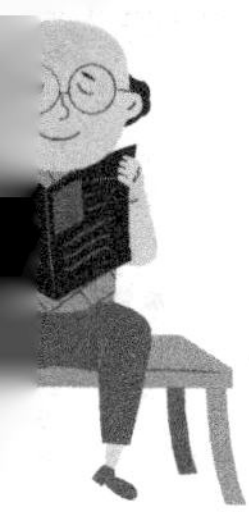

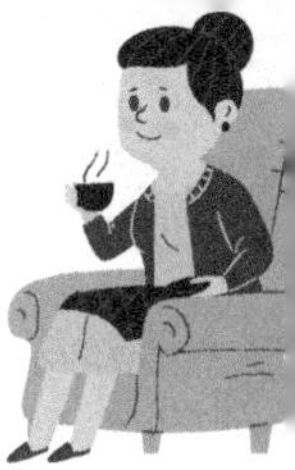

Castle Visit

It was a beautiful autumn day when the elderly couple Walter and Edith decided to visit the famous castle in their town. They had often heard about the majestic structure, but they had never had the opportunity to explore it themselves.

As they entered the castle, they were greeted by a friendly museum guide who told them about the rich history of the castle. He spoke of times past, of knights in shining armor, of booming cannons, and fearsome attacks. Walter and Edith listened with fascination as they were led through the impressive halls and corridors of the castle.

They learned about the epic battles that were once fought around the castle, and of the brave men and women who defended it. They saw the ancient weapons and armor still hanging on the walls of the castle, and imagined the heroic stories they could tell.

The museum guide then led them to the secret passages and hidden rooms of the castle.

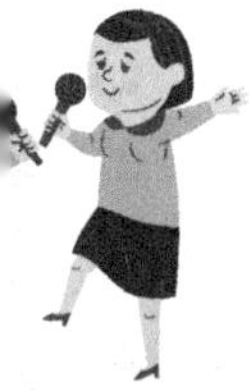

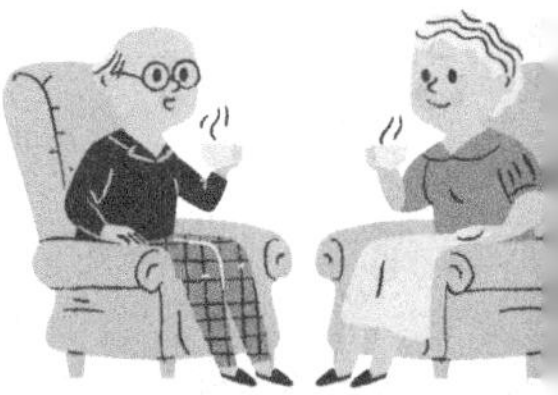

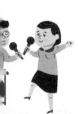
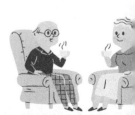

Walter and Edith were amazed by the ingenious construction and clever tricks that the castle's inhabitants had once used to outwit their enemies. They heard about the conditions in the castle, about the hard but fulfilling lives of the people who lived there.

They saw the old kitchens and pantries, the bedrooms and workspaces, and imagined the bustling, lively life that once took place in these rooms.

The museum guide also led them through the beautiful castle garden, still filled with carefully tended roses and other flowers. Walter and Edith enjoyed the freshness of the air and the beauty of nature, reminiscing about the many happy hours they had spent in their own gardens.

To conclude the tour, they visited the old dungeon of the castle, a gloomy yet fascinating place.

They heard about the unfortunate souls who were once imprisoned there, and the secrets that these ancient walls still concealed.

The visit to the castle was a journey into the past for Walter and Edith. It stirred up many memories and emotions in them, allowing them to appreciate the history and heritage of their city in a new and vibrant way.

As they left the castle, they felt fulfilled and grateful. They had not only learned more about the history and culture of their hometown but also gathered valuable shared memories that they would always cherish in their hearts. They were happy to have spent this day together and looked forward to many more adventures ahead.

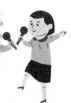

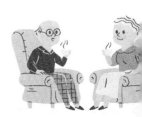

The New Family

Johann and Emma, an honest and lovable couple from a small village in USA, wished for nothing more than to experience the joy of parenthood. They had been trying to start a family for years, but after a series of disappointing news from doctors, their long-cherished dream seemed unreachable. Emma fell into a sad silence, finding no solace in her usual life and spending her days alone in their small, cozy farmhouse.

However, Johann, a man of unwavering optimism and love, did not give up hope. He spent long nights scouring adoption agencies across the country, hoping to find a child to whom they could offer a loving home. After months of calls, letters, and sleepless nights, Johann came across a photo of a little girl named Elena, who lived in a crowded orphanage far away. When Emma saw Elena's picture with her rosy cheeks and bright eyes, she felt a wave of warmth and hope in her heart.

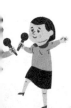
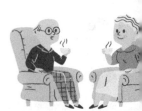

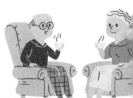

The social worker's conviction that they would be suitable parents was a challenge - home visits were conducted, inspections and interviews were held. Emma and Johann provided every conceivable piece of information about their lives, their farm, their ties to the community, and much more, to prove that they could offer Elena the loving and secure home she deserved.

Finally, the long-awaited call came - they had been approved. The journey to Elena was a whirlwind of nervousness and excitement. Would Elena like her new room, which they had lovingly decorated with toys and books? What if Elena had difficulty adjusting to her new home?

As the couple stepped out of the car in front of the orphanage, Emma trembled with excitement. But as Elena approached them and whispered shyly, "Mom?" Emma was overwhelmed by a wave of love. In that moment, she knew that her family, just as she had always imagined it, was finally complete.

The formalities passed like a dream, and before they knew it, Elena was safely and happily seated in her car seat as they drove towards their new home. Together, they admired the picturesque landscape passing by her window.

In the first night, Emma lay awake, watching Elena sleep in her cradle. Every breath Elena took was a sign of hope and joy for Emma. And so began the years of happiness - the first steps, words, and birthdays.

Summers were filled with adventures on the farm, picking berries, and swimming trips to the nearby lake.

Winters were a time of cuddling and laughter, marked by baking days, snowmen, and Johann's storytelling by the fireplace.

School days brought colorful autumn walks, lovingly prepared packed lunches, and homework assistance. Holidays and family gatherings were times of laughter and love as they watched Elena grow into a wonderful young woman.

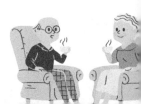

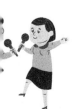
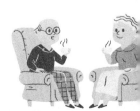

Today, Emma looks proudly at her daughter, who has grown into a smart, curious, and loving young woman. She is surrounded by a community that has celebrated every step of her journey. Despite all the previous challenges, Elena has brought joy and fulfillment to her life that surpasses anything they could have ever imagined.

In Search of Happiness

In a small, peaceful town once lived a man named William. William led a simple life, yet he yearned for something he defined as "true happiness." One day, he decided it was time to embark on a quest.

William's first stop on his journey was the big city. He had heard that happiness could be found amidst the hustle and bustle of urban life. He found employment, enjoyed the nightlife, and met many interesting people. However, despite all the new experiences, William didn't truly feel happy. So, he moved on, this time to a picturesque village by the sea. He thought that happiness might be found in the tranquility and beauty of nature. He spent his days taking walks on the beach and relishing the peaceful atmosphere. Yet, even here, though he appreciated the beauty and serenity of the place, he didn't feel fulfilled.

His next stop was a monastery high in the mountains. He hoped that happiness might be found in spirituality and inner peace.

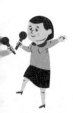
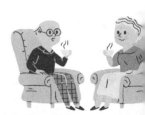

He meditated, read spiritual texts, and engaged in lengthy conversations with the monks. But even here, he couldn't find the true happiness he was searching for. Disappointed and somewhat desperate, William returned to his hometown. He was discouraged and believed that he might never find true happiness.

One day, while strolling through the familiar streets of his city, he ran into an old friend. They decided to have a coffee together in a nearby café. They reminisced about old times, laughed over shared memories, and exchanged stories.

As they talked and laughed, William noticed a warm, pleasant feeling in his heart. He felt happy, fulfilled, and content. He realized that he hadn't found true happiness in the bustle of the city, the tranquility of the sea, or the spirituality of the monastery, but here, in the simple joy of a good conversation with an old friend.

He had come to understand that true happiness is not something to seek and find, but something that already exists within us.

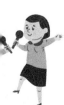

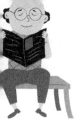

It's the joy in the little things in life, the love for our friends and family, and the memories and experiences we gather on our life journey.

William had completed his journey and found true happiness. And it wasn't in an exotic location or in a deep spiritual experience, but in his own heart, surrounded by the people and memories he loved.

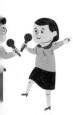

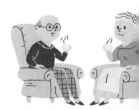

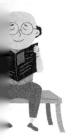
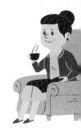

A Picnic Journey

Once, in a small town called Lowforest, lived a kind-hearted elderly gentleman named Mr. Meyer. Every year, when spring arrived and the flowers began to bloom, Mr. Meyer would have a traditional picnic in the local park, a tradition he inherited from his parents.

On this particular spring day, Mr. Meyer packed his basket with all his favorite foods: homemade potato salad following his mother's recipe, freshly baked rolls from the bakery around the corner, and strawberry cake, which his wife used to love. He also took his old blanket, which had survived many years and picnics.

With his picnic basket and blanket, he made his way to the park. As he entered the park, he could hear the laughter of children playing on the playground. He remembered the times when he brought his own children to play in the park. A smile spread across his face as he relived those sweet memories.

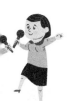
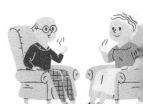

He chose a spot under a large, shade-giving tree, beneath which he and his wife had often enjoyed their picnics. As he spread out the blanket, he reminisced about the many afternoons they had spent there, telling stories, laughing, and forgetting the world around them.

While eating his potato salad, he recalled the many family picnics they had hosted in this park. The memory of his children's laughter, the delicious food, and the loving company of his wife warmed his heart.

After the meal, he leaned back and watched the clouds drift by. He remembered the many cloud shapes he and his children had seen, and how they told stories about the forms they saw in the clouds.

As the day dwindled, Mr. Meyer packed up his belongings and began the journey home. He felt fulfilled and happy to have relived these precious memories. Even though times had changed, the memories continued to live on in his heart.

Mr. Meyer's story reminds us that memories are a precious gift that we always carry with us.

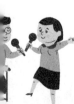

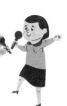

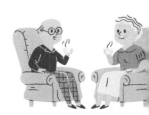

They remind us of life's joys and bring smiles to our faces, even when the people and places that created them are no longer with us. Every time we recall these times, they continue to live on in our hearts, bringing us joy and comfort.

Made in the USA
Columbia, SC
05 May 2025